BRITISH
MEDICAL BULLETIN

VOLUME FORTY-FIVE
1989

The colour printing in this issue
was sponsored by the
SPECIAL CARDIAC FUND,
BROMPTON HOSPITAL

CHURCHILL LIVINGSTONE
EDINBURGH, LONDON, MELBOURNE AND NEW YORK

CHURCHILL LIVINGSTONE
Medical Division of Longman Group UK Limited

Distributed in the United States of America by Churchill
Livingstone Inc., 1560 Broadway, New York, NY 10036, and
by associated companies, branches and representatives
throughout the world.

ISSN 0007-1420
ISBN 0 443 04200 4

BRITISH MEDICAL BULLETIN

British Medical Bulletin is published four times each year, in January, April, July and October.

Subscriptions and single-copy orders should be sent to: Longman Group UK Ltd, Subscriptions Department, Fourth Avenue, Harlow, Essex CM19 5AA.

Subscription rates for 1990 are: £80 (UK) or £96.00/$165.00 (overseas)

Single copies will be available at £25.00 (UK) or £31.50/$49.25 (overseas)

NEXT ISSUE

CHURCHILL LIVINGSTONE, Medical Division of Longman Group U.K. Limited. Typeset and printed by H Charlesworth & Co Ltd, Huddersfield

Distributed in the United States of America by Churchill Livingstone Inc., 1560 Broadway, New York, NY 10036, and by associated companies, branches and representatives throughout the world. This journal is indexed, abstracted and/or publishd online in the following media: Current Contents, Scientific Serials Review, Excerpta Medica, USSR Academy of Science, Biological Abstracts, UMI (Microform), BRS Colleague (full text), Index Medicus, BIOSIS, NMLUIS, Adonis

© The British Council 1989

ISSN 0007-1420   **ISBN 0 443 04200 4**

Non-invasive Cardiac Imaging

Scientific Editor: *D G Gibson*

1989 Vol. 45 No. 4

Dr D G Gibson chaired the committee which included Professor P N T Wells and Mr D B Longmore that planned this number of the *British Medical Bulletin*. We are grateful to them for their help, and particularly to Dr Gibson who acted as Scientific Editor for the number.

British Medical Bulletin is published by Churchill Livingstone for The British Council, 10 Spring Gardens, London SW1A 2BN

British Medical Bulletin (1989) Vol. 45, No. 4, pp. i–ii
© The British Council 1989

Introduction

D G Gibson
Brompton Hospital, London, UK

It is only a little over twenty years ago that the word 'non-invasive' was introduced to describe a group of methods used to study left ventricular function based on external graphical recordings. The term was chosen to distinguish them from those based on cardiac catheterisation, then the dominant diagnostic method in cardiology. At first the contribution of these new methods was small, but progress has been rapid and the balance has been profoundly altered, first by the appearance of M-mode echocardiography, and more recently by the imaging methods with which this volume of the BMB is concerned. Over the same period, invasive investigation has changed little, so that, with the conspicuous exception of coronary artery anatomy, virtually every cardiac diagnosis previously made by cardiac catheterisation can now be made noninvasively.

These new methods have also made new information accessible. Echocardiography delineates valve anatomy in detail, and in complex congenital heart disease, relations between valve cusps and great arteries, as well as tensor apparatus to ventricular myocardium can be studied in detail. Complex flow patterns within ventricles and through or around normal or prosthetic valves can be mapped by colour flow Doppler or magnetic resonance imaging. Most significant of all, perhaps, is the ability to study myocardium: its thickness, wall dynamics, perfusion, metabolism and constitution by these new techniques used in combination.

Not only are these new methods more comprehensive than many based on catheterisation, but they can be applied more widely to normal populations, or those at risk, particularly to those suspected of having coronary artery disease. Normal aging, for example, is now known to have major effects on diastolic function or the response of ejection fraction to exercise. Groups of patients can be identified noninvasively as being of high risk of having significant coronary artery disease, with correspondingly impaired prognosis, so that expensive invasive methods can be used with more discrimination.

Diagnosis on its own, however accurate it may be, is of no direct

0007–1420/89/0045–i/$10.00

benefit to a patient. Benefit comes only when increased information is translated into better management. Echocardiography has had a major impact in reducing the need for cardiac catheterisation in patients with complex congenital heart disease: in those with total anomalous pulmonary venous drainage, for example, operative results have improved strikingly when the depressant effects of contrast angiographic media are avoided. The same applies to the large majority of those with valvular heart disease.

It is with these new methods, and their clinical and research potiental that the present BMB is concerned. They are the fruit of developing technology, particularly of newer methods of digital image processing. Chapters have therefore been provided outlining their technical basis, stressing their limitations as well as their potential. Later sections describe how nuclear methods can be used to study right and left ventricular wall motion, and myocardial perfusion and metabolism. The use of echocardiography in congenital and valvular heart disease, and in assessing ventricular function is outlined, and the additional contribution of colour flow mapping described. Magnetic resonance imaging is covered in some detail, to show how this new method can be used to study anatomy, flow, and tissue characterisation, and a final section gives early results of fast CT, another promising imaging method. Taken together, these chapters have been written to give an idea of the scope of these methods, to summarise the present position, and to introduce the ideas, and the literature on which they are based to anyone newly entering the field, either as a clinician or research worker. It seems likely that the future progress of cardiology will be closely determined by the development of these methods and by the new information and ideas that they provide.

British Medical Bulletin (1989) Vol. 45, No. 4, pp. 829–837
© The British Council 1989

Technical introduction to echocardiography

P N T Wells
Department of Medical Physics and University Department of Radiodiagnosis, Bristol General Hospital, Bristol

Pulse-echo ultrasound can be used to measure distance along a narrow beam with resolution limited by the wavelength and, ultimately, by attenuation. Time-position (M-mode) recording can be used to study structure motion. Real-time two-dimensional imaging can be achieved with mechanical scanning or electronically controlled phase array transducers, the frame rate being limited by the depth of penetration and the image line density. Blood flow can be detected by the Doppler effect. Continuous wave Doppler systems lack depth discrimination, but this can be provided by pulsed Doppler although range-velocity ambiguities may occur. Blood flow volume rate can be estimated from measurements of velocity and area; the simultaneous use of wide and narrow beams reduces the errors. Duplex scanning uses two-dimensional real-time imaging for Doppler sample volume localization. Two-dimensional colour-coded images of blood flow can be produced in real time. Endoscopic scanning avoids problems due to bone and gas. Contrast agents can be used to enhance the echogenicity of blood.

Echocardiography owes its origin to the work of Inge Edler and Helmuth Hertz in the 1950s. It was they who demonstrated the relationships between ultrasonic echoes and the structure and function of the heart.[1] In the thirty-five years that have passed since their pioneering research, remarkable progress has been made, beginning with the widespread acceptance of M-mode studies, followed by real-time imaging, Doppler and duplex techniques, and culminating in the recent excitement of colour-coded Doppler imaging.

0007–1420/89/0045–0829/$10.00

In comparison with other methods of studying the heart, ultrasound has the advantage of combining real-time two-dimensional imaging and the measurement of blood flow velocity with non-invasive and apparently completely safe techniques. Additional information can be obtained by the minimally-intrusive endoscopic approach and by the use of vascular contrast agents. Indeed, were it not for the constraints imposed by overlying gas and bone, and the range-velocity ambiguity of pulsed Doppler detection, ultrasound would likely be the ideal method for examining the heart. Moreover, the equipment is relatively inexpensive.

PULSE-ECHO ULTRASOUND

Ultrasound consists of mechanical vibrations, the frequencies of which are so high that they are above the range of human hearing. In echocardiography, frequencies in the range 1–15 MHz (million cycles per second) are employed; the corresponding range of wavelengths is 1.5–0.1 mm in soft tissues, in which ultrasound travels at a speed of about 1500 m s^{-1}. At these frequencies, ultrasound is generated and detected by transducers using piezoelectric materials which convert electrical energy to ultrasound and vice versa.[2] Transducers with apertures of a centimetre or so can produce quite narrow beams of ultrasound, which can be both focused and pulsed.

Because there are only small differences in the speeds of ultrasound in different tissues, the distance travelled by a pulse of ultrasound is proportional to time and the beam can be assumed to be straight. The small differences in the speeds, and the different densities of different tissues, combine to result in differences in characteristic impedance, however, and when an ultrasonic pulse meets boundaries between different tissues a small amount is reflected.[3] (Almost complete reflexion takes place at boundaries between soft tissue and either gas or bone, because of the very large acoustic impedance differences.) The detection of the resulting echoes allows the positions of the corresponding reflectors (or small scatterers) on the ultrasonic beam axis to be determined. The pulse-echo go-and-return delay time is about 1.33 µs per mm.

The spatial resolution of an ultrasonic pulse-echo imaging system is determined by the cross-sectional dimensions of the ultrasonic beam and the length of the ultrasonic pulse. Ultimately, these both depend on the ultrasonic wavelength: the resolution becomes better as the wavelength is reduced. Of course, the wavelength is inversely proportional to the frequency and so increasing the frequency improves the resolution. Unfortunately, the attenuation of ultrasound also increases with frequency,[3] and this means that decreasing echo amplitude limits the maximum frequency that can result in detectable echo signals from any given depth.

In order to compensate for the relatively high attenuation of echoes from deeper structures, the amplification provided by the ultrasonic receiver is arranged to increase with time following the transmission of the ultrasonic pulse. This process, known as time-gain-control (TGC), can usually be adjusted by the operator to provide the optimum display.

The time delay between the transmission of an ultrasonic pulse and the reception of the echo from the maximum depth of interest determines the maximum pulse repetition frequency. For example, for a depth of 150 mm this time is 200 μs, corresponding to a maximum PRF of 5000 per second.

TIME-POSITION RECORDING: THE M-MODE

A time-position recording (an M-mode display) can be obtained as shown in Figure 1. The sweep time of the slow-speed timebase is typically about 3 s, allowing a few cardiac cycles to be displayed. For detailed study and quantitative analysis, a continuous hard-copy recording of the M-mode display is required. Such a tracing can be made using a fibre-optic ultraviolet recorder, or a thermal printer.

M-mode recordings allow cardiac structure motion to be quantified in terms of amplitude and velocity.[4] Additional information can be obtained by the simultaneous recording of ECG and PCG signals, especially when valve function timing is of interest.

REAL-TIME TWO-DIMENSIONAL SCANNING

The production of an image of a cross-section through the scanned anatomy is accomplished by relating the positions of registrations on the display to the positions of the corresponding echo-producing structure within a defined two-dimensional plane in the patient.[3] To be useful in studying the heart, imaging has to be performed in real time.

The ultrasonic beam can be mechanically or electrically scanned, as illustrated in Figure 2. For examining the heart, the

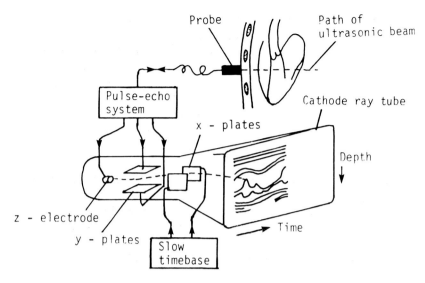

Fig. 1. M-mode system for time-position recording of structure motion. The z-electrode controls the brightness of the display according to the echo amplitude; the x- and y-plates respectively control the horizontal and vertical deflexions of the electron beam, which is shown as a dotted line within the cathode ray tube.

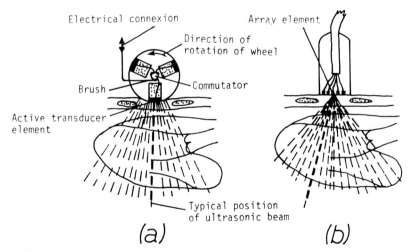

Fig. 2. Real-time two-dimensional scanning systems. (**a**) Mechanical sector scanner. As each element in turn sweeps through a sector within the patient (through a stationary acoustic window, not shown in the diagram), the commutator and brush connect it to the electronic system. (**b**) Phased array sector scanner.

sector format is ideal because it allows the maximum area to be visualized through the narrow windows between the ribs and lungs. With mechanical scanning, the transducer can conveniently be fabricated as a disk or as an annular array, can the electronic circuitry can be quite simple.[5] Nowadays, however, phased array sector scanning is almost always used for echocardiography because of the lightness and convenience of the probe and the versatility of ultrasonic beam control that it makes possible.[5] Moreover, the falling cost of electronic systems allows increasingly useful features to be provided for similar amounts of money.

In a phased array system, the rectangular transducer consists of a large number of narrow strips of piezoelectric material, each with a separate electrical connexion. Each transducer element can be considered to radiate a cylindrical wavelet of ultrasound and to be, in the plane of the scan, an omnidirectional receiver. If all the elements are excited simultaneously, the transducer behaves like a rectangular plate and the beam direction is perpendicular to the face of the probe. If the elements are excited sequentially across the array, however, the surface tangential to the cylindrical wavelets travels away from the probe at an angle with respect to the geometrical central axis, dependent on the time delays across the array. Thus, the beam can be steered in any direction within a sector by appropriate choice of these time delays. Moreover, the beam can be electronically focused at any chosen depth. Likewise, the receiving beam can be steered by variable delay lines in the receiver, except that there is the additional capability of sweeping the position of the focus along the beam so that it remains in focus along the entire beam length.

The image frame rate determines the speed of structure motion that can be studied in real-time scanning systems. Assuming a typical PRF of 5000 per second, 5000 lines of image information can be collected each second. If an image frame with satisfactory spatial information can be formed by, for example, 200 lines, then the frame rate is 25 per second. Thus it is necessary to compromise between frame rate and line density.

Real-time images can be studied in real time, or they may be recorded on video tape for subsequent review. Systems designed for echocardiography usually also have 'frame freeze' facilities which allow images, or short series of images, to be stored in memory for immediate review and for hard-copy recording, either on photographic film or thermal printer. The ECG is usually simultaneously recorded for time correlation.

DOPPLER ULTRASOUND

The frequency of a reflected ultrasonic wave is equal to that of the incident wave if the reflector is stationary. Movement of the reflector towards the source, however, results in compression of the wavelength (and a corresponding increase in frequency), and vice versa. The phenomenon is called the Doppler effect.[6] For reflectors moving with velocities commonly occurring in the body, and with ultrasound in the low megahertz frequency range, the difference in frequency between the received and transmitted waves generally lies in the audible range. For example, with a reflector velocity of 100 mm s^{-1} and an ultrasonic frequency of 3 MHz, the Doppler shift frequency is 400 Hz. It is the component of velocity along the ultrasonic beam axis that determines the frequency shift; the calculated shift frequency has to be multiplied by the cosine of the angle between the direction of movement and that of the ultrasonic beam if the two are not coincident. Thus, in principle no Doppler shift is detected when the motion is perpendicular to the beam.

The simplest Doppler systems use continuous wave ultrasound and so they cannot separate moving targets according to their depths along the ultrasound beam although they can distinguish between approaching and receding reflectors, or between forward and reverse flow directions.[5] Range selectivity can be obtained, however, by pulsing the ultrasonic transmitter and 'gating' the receiver at the time delay corresponding to the depth of the sample volume of interest.[5]

For blood flow studies, the choice of ultrasonic frequency is determined by the compromise between the reflectivity of blood and the attenuation in overlying tissues, both of which increase with increasing frequency. For intracardiac blood flow investigations, 3 MHz is usually about the optimum. There is, however, a further important limitation in the performance of pulsed Doppler systems. If the Doppler shift frequency exceeds half the pulse repetition frequency, the signal is inadequately sampled and the estimation of the shift frequency is ambiguous; the so-called 'Nyquist limit' is exceeded and aliasing occurs in the output signal. Because the maximum PRF is determined by the depth (or range) of the required penetration, this gives rise to the 'range-velocity' limit. If, for example, the target of interest is the one which has the highest velocity, the problem can be avoided by increasing the PRF above that corresponding to the maximum target depth, but the data then need to be interpreted thoughtfully.

Much useful information can be obtained by listening to the Doppler signals. For quantitative analysis, however, it is necessary to determine the instantaneous maximum or mean frequencies, or the time-varying distribution of the full frequency spectrum. If the blood flow velocity corresponding to the average instantaneous mean frequency is multiplied by the vessel cross-sectional area, the blood flow volume rate can be derived although it is important to remember that incomplete or non-uniform insonation of the flowing blood leads to errors for which correction may be difficult.[7] In some situations, such as in the ascending aorta viewed from the suprasternal notch, this problem may be avoided by simultaneous insonation with wide and narrow beams; the Doppler power spectra then allow the volume flow rate to be derived without the need to know either the cross-sectional area of the vessel or the vector direction of flow.[8]

DUPLEX SCANNING

The combination of real-time imaging with Doppler flow velocity measurement is the basis of the duplex scanner. The real-time image is used to locate regions of interest, within which the Doppler sample volume is positioned. Referring to Figure 2, typical ultrasonic beam positions are indicated; the sample volume could be located anywhere along these beams, allowing flow in the corresponding regions to be assessed. The Doppler system may use the same transducer as the imager, or a separate transducer with independent within-plane directional control may be provided. If the same transducer is used for imaging and for Doppler, simultaneous operation is possible with a phased array (because the direction of the beam can be changed instantaneously) but not with a mechanical scanner.[5] Separate transducers allow different but optimum ultrasonic frequencies to be used for imaging and Doppler, but a compromise is needed if the same transducer is used for both purposes.

The length of the pulsed Doppler sample volume can be adjusted to match the clinical situation, and the relative directions of the ultrasonic beam and the flow can usually be determined. Thus, qualitative results can often be obtained in the assessment of intracardiac flow velocities.[5]

COLOUR-CODED DOPPLER IMAGING

Figure 3 shows how two-dimensional real-time imaging producing a grey-scale representation of an anatomical cross-section can be combined with a real-time image in which Doppler flow signals are displayed in colour. The method depends on fast signal processing,[9] but nevertheless there is a fundamental limitation on the maximum image frame rate. The proportion of the time occupied by real-time pulse-echo imaging is relatively short; for Doppler imaging, it is necessary for each image line to be stationary for enough time to allow the measurement of the lowest Doppler shift frequency necessary to establish the corresponding flow conditions. Typically, the maximum image frame rate for a complete 50° sector is around 5 per second; in modern instruments, the frame rate is increased by narrowing the colour-coded sector angle, increasing the low-frequency Doppler-shift threshold and interpolating between sparsely-sampled lines.[9]

In echocardiography, the image is usually colour-coded according to the Doppler shift frequency using a yellow–red–black–navy-blue scale. Black corresponds to zero vector velocity; yellow may be for forward flow, blue for reverse, or vice versa. Flow disturbance, which results in Doppler frequency spectral broadening, may be coded in a contrasting colour, such as green. Aliasing as a result of exceeding the Nyquist limit is usually self-

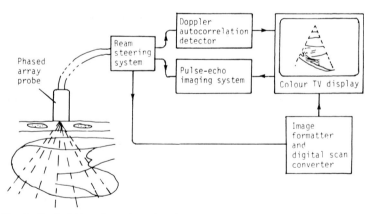

Fig. 3. Typical Doppler colour flow imaging system. The phased array probe produces a grey-scale real-time pulse-echo sector scan, under the control of the beam steering system, the image formatter and digital scan converter. Simultaneously, the Doppler autocorrelation flow detector colour codes the two-dimensional image according to the flow velocity vectors in the scanned sector.

evident through obviously artifactual localized reversal of the colour scale. In interpreting colour flow images, directional information often needs careful consideration of the vector directions of the local ultrasonic beam and the flow pattern.

ENDOSCOPIC METHODS

Ultrasonic access ot the heart can easily be obtained by a transducer mounted on an endoscope introduced into the oesophagus. Using this approach, excellent cross-sectional and Doppler studies are possible without problems due to intervening tissues, gas or bone.[10]

CONTRAST AGENTS

Gas bubbles encapsulated in soluble microspheres greatly enhance the echogenicity of blood when administered intra-arterially or intravenously. Bubbles which are small enough to cross through the lungs are beginning to become available.[11] The use of such agents is already showing promise for the detection of small intracardiac shunts and valvular leaks, and for tissue characterization of the myocardium and the assessment of perfusion defects.

REFERENCES

1 Edler I, Hertz CH. The use of the ultrasonic reflectoscope for the continuous recording of the movements of heart walls. K fysiogr Sällsk Lund Forh 1954; 24: 40–58
2 Hunt JW, Arditi M, Foster MS. Ultrasound transducers for pulse-echo medical imaging. IEEE Trans Biomed Eng 1983; BME-30: 453–481
3 Wells PNT. Biomedical ultrasonics. London: Academic Press, 1977
4 Feigenbaum H. Echocardiography. Philadelphia: Lea and Febiger, 1972
5 Wells PNT. Instrumentation. In: Taylor KJW, Burns PN, Wells PNT, eds. Clinical applications of Doppler ultrasound. New York: Raven Press, 1988: p. 26
6 Wells PNT. Basic principles and Doppler physics. In: Taylor KJW, Burns PN, Wells PNT, eds. Clinical applications of Doppler ultrasound. New York: Raven Press, 1988: p. 1
7 Gill RW. Measurement of blood flow by ultrasound: accuracy and sources of error. Ultrasound Med Biol 1985; 11: 625–641
8 Evans JM, Skidmore, R, Baker JD, Wells PNT. A new approach to the noninvasive measurement of cardiac output using an annular array technique. II: Practical implementation and results. Ultrasound Med Biol 1989; 15: 179–187
9 Wells PNT. Doppler ultrasound in medical diagnosis. Br J Radiol 1989; 62: 399–420
10 Roelandt JRTC, Sutherland GR. Oesophageal echocardiography. Br Heart J 1988; 60: 1–3
11 Miszalok V, Fritzsch T, Schartl M. Myocardial perfusion defects in contrast echocardiology: spectral and temporal localisation. Ultrasound Med Biol 1986; 12: 581–586

British Medical Bulletin (1989) Vol. 45, No. 4, pp. 838–847
© The British Council 1989

Technical introduction to nuclear imaging

D S Dymond
St Bartholomew's Hospital, London

It is very important to pay attention to technical detail when acquiring nuclear scans of the heart. It must be remembered that not only is the heart a three dimensional structure, which imposes its own limitations on the interpretation of information represented as two dimensional images, but the organ also moves which will in turn degrade static images. Dynamic studies of left ventricular function must be able to resolve the rapidly changing events of the cardiac cycle which makes specific technical demands upon the imaging equipment and computer system used. In spite of these potential drawbacks, both static and dynamic imaging of the heart using radiopharmaceuticals are widely used in a clinical and research environment. In this article some of the technical considerations will be covered as they apply to both the commonly used clinical applications of nuclear cardiology and some of the newer but potentially exciting techniques will also be covered briefly.

RADIOPHARMACEUTICALS FOR CARDIOVASCULAR NUCLEAR MEDICINE

Most readers will be familiar with thallium-201 and technetium-99m as the two most commonly used radionuclides in nuclear cardiology. It is however helpful to consider the radiopharmaceuticals in groups — (A) the infarct avid agents, (B) agents for myocardial perfusion scanning, (C) metabolic tracers, (D) labelled cardiac antibodies and catecholamine analogues, and (E) agents for cardiac function studies. Description in detail is beyond the scope of this article but an up to date comprehensive review can be found by Elmaleh and colleagues.[1]

0007–1420/89/0045–0838/$10.00

INFARCT AVID IMAGING

This term is used to describe a technique whereby acutely necrotic myocardium is imaged by the administration of a tracer which delineates the necrotic area as increased uptake rather than as an image defect. This is sometimes known as a 'hot spot scan'. This was evaluated in detail in the 1970s when it was discovered that bone scanning agents such as stannous pyrophosphate and other related compounds, when labelled with technetium-99m, could demonstrate acute myocardial infarction.[2] The technical demands for producing images are small and analogue images could be obtained with conventional gamma camera systems even without a computer. A very high correlation rate was obtained between the site of the tracer uptake and corresponding electrocardiographic Q waves. The images could be interpreted qualitatively in polaroid or X-ray format. Non Q wave infarctions tended to produce diffuse uptake in a substantial number of patients and in addition many people with unstable angina showed scintigraphic evidence of necrosis despite having normal enzymes. This technique, however, offers little in most patients with acute infarction where the diagnosis is apparent from clinical, electrocardiographic and enzymatic data. Occasionally in patients with equivocal enzymes or those with left bundle branch block or permanent pacemakers *in situ* the scans could provide relevant information, not otherwise available. Sizing an acute myocardial infarction by the area of uptake of isotope is more difficult, especially as the images are two dimensional representing a 3 dimensional event. Single photon emission computerised tomography (SPECT), which is further discussed below has led to an improved assessment of infarct size.[3] The main problem with the technique for this purpose, however, is that the scans do not become positive for about 24–48 hours after the event by which time in modern cardiological practice any intervention to salvage myocardium should have taken place.

More recently the monoclonal antibody antimyosin has been produced which, when labelled with indium-111, produces images as the antimyosin antiody tags on to free myosin which is exposed after myocardial cell lysis. The drawback of the technique is extensive blood pool contamination with indium and the fact that this isotope is not as good as an imaging agent as technetium. The latter is really ideal for gamma camera studies because of its single energy peak at 140 keV. Again with the antimyosin images the

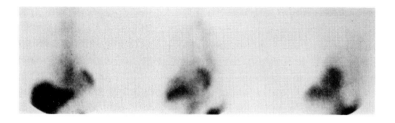

Fig. 1 Indium-111 labelled antimyosin images 48 hours after injection in a patient with extensive anterior and lateral myocardial infarction. Images are anteroposterior (left), 40° left anterior oblique (middle) and 70° left anterior oblique. Dense uptake in the liver is seen but myocardial uptake in the anterolateral wall is evident on the anteroposterior image and extensive posterolateral uptake on the two left anterior oblique images. The radiopharmaceutical is taken up by necrotic myocardium.

scans are at their best approximately 48 hours after the acute event (Fig. 1). The main advantage of antimyosin over the organic phosphates is that their delivery is not dependent on residual flow. Thus with pyrophosphate it was possible to have negative scans if there was no flow in the centre of the infarct and this is not something routinely seen with antimyosin. It is unlikely that antimyosin will revolutionize the practice of medicine in ischaemic heart disease for the same reason that pyrophosphate did not. However the experience with myocardial necrosis during rejection episodes in the transplanted heart suggest that antimyosin may well have an important role to play here,[4] as well as perhaps in acute myocarditis.

MYOCARDIAL PERFUSION IMAGING

Thallium-201 is a monovalent cation which is an analogue of potassium and, when injected intravenously, distributes around the body in proportion to regional cardiac output. This is true both from organ to organ and for different areas within an organ. Thus when thallium-201 distributes in the myocardium and joins the potassium pool, images may be produced which represent regional myocardial perfusion at the time the tracer was distributing. Thallium has monopolized the myocardial perfusion market since the early 1970s and superseded agents such as potassium-43. A resting myocardial perfusion scan in a normal heart should show homogeneous uptake of the tracer and in the presence of scar tissue secondary to myocardial infarction an image defect will be present. Thus abnormal ares are shown as image defects or 'cold spots'. The initial excitement about the potential use of this technique to screen patients with chest pain in casualty departments to decide whether they had infarcted or not soon waned, as the presence of a defect on any day cannot tell one whether this is scar tissue or reversibly ischaemic tissue and nor can the infarct be dated. The main use of perfusion scanning is as an adjunct to exercise testing where 2 mCi of the tracer (74 mbq) are injected intravenously, preferably into an elbow vein, at the peak of a treadmill exercise test. The isotope distributes into the myocardium and areas that have been rendered ischaemic by the exercise test will show up as defects. Imaging is carried out, starting about 5 minutes after the injection and peak myocardial levels usually occur at about ten minutes after injection. Conventionally three or four views are taken using a standard gamma camera and the anteroposterior, 30° and 60° left anterior oblique are the most commonly ones used. We have in the past utilized a left lateral in addition although attenuation of the isotope often makes this particular view difficult to interpret. Because thallium has a low energy (80 keV) there is a lot of attenuation and scatter by the tissues between the myocardium and gamma camera crystal. Cameras have been specially designed for use with thallium and their crystals are usually only a $\frac{1}{4}$ of an inch thick. The collimator used is usually low energy all purpose (LEAP). The low energy of the isotope means that images are always likely to be of low resolution and in addition the thallium is distributed elsewhere in the body, not just to the heart. There is thus a lot of background extra cardiac activity and it is the liver, stomach and spleen which tend to interfere most with the cardiac images, particularly with the inferior wall. One normally collects about 300,000 counts per view in the heart itself and some workers put a lead apron over the abdomen to shield the splanchnic viscera and hence exclude photons from there from the images. Splanchnic counts can be minimized by imaging the patient in the fasting state. Following the collection of the exercise data the patient is asked to return 4–6 hours later for a repeat series of images. After this time 'redistribution' will have taken place and thallium will have washed into areas that were ischaemic and under perfused and out of areas that were normally perfused. By comparing the delayed images to the immediate post exercise ones regions which were ischaemic during exercise and which were normal at rest can be visualized. Areas that show no redistribution between post exercise and delayed images are often labelled as infarcts or scars and certainly areas with electrocardiographic Q waves do show this pattern. However in some cases failure of redistribution at 6 hours may reflect severe ischaemia without actual infarction and if the ECG does not show Q waves in the corresponding areas it is prudent to re-image the patient at rest 24 hours later or even by a separate thallium injection at rest a week or so later.

The interpretation of the images requires great practice and expertise. Because of their low resolution nature it is important that the images should be processed with a computer and this includes background correction and smoothing.[5] Some quantification technique should be used and these are too numerous to mention in this article but include assessment of circumferential profiles or washout rates. The exact details of this are beyond the scope of this article, and the reader is referred to a chapter by Maddahi et al.[6] The amount of lung uptake of thallium on the images has also proved useful as increased lung uptake seems to correlate with raised left ventricular end diastolic pressure on exercise and may reflect more severe global ischaemia.[7] Attempts to quantify the amount of coronary artery disease into single, double or triple vessel disease, or to predict left main stem disease have not proved successful with any degree of confidence.

Gating the thallium images to the electrocardiographic signal overcomes motion artefact and improves the resolution of the images. However the trade off is that the time for each image to be acquired increases significantly if enough counts are to be achieved, and it must be remembered that redistribution of the tracer starts as soon as ischaemia subsides. Therefore if the image acquisition is too long one may have already entered the redistribution phase and reduced the diagnostic capability of the images. Tomographic imaging is described later in this article.

Despite all its drawbacks, namely its long half-life of 72 hours, its poor energy for gamma camera imaging, the non-physiological nature of the isotope and the difficulty with image quantification, thallium scanning has been remarkably successful in clarification of equivocal exercise tests and appears to be of great value in predicting prognosis in coronary disease. It is also used, although less frequently, in non-coronary conditions, for example right ventricular hypertrophy can be assessed by the appearance of the right ventricle on a resting scan and it has also been used in conditions such as sarcoidosis. The drawbacks in the radiopharmaceutical have prompted the search for a technetium based compound to replace it. Several of these compounds are under investigation and the most widely studied are the group known as the isonitriles of which MIBI has been the one most extensively evaluated.[8] This is not a monovalent cation and so once injected does not redistribute within the potassium pool like thallium. In order to image at rest and exercise MIBI must be injected on the 2 separate occasions, usually 24 hours apart. This of course is a major drawback particularly if patients live some way from the imaging centre, as the whole sequence cannot be completed on one visit. There are also some doubts as to whether these agents faithfully reproduce perfusion and liver uptake is still proving a problem. Plate 1 is an example of a technetium labelled MIBI scan at rest and on exercise on separate days from a patient with coronary artery disease. The better imaging quality of technetium has certainly made these images more attractive to look at, although quantification has not yet been evaluated properly. It is quite likely that within the next few years thallium will be replaced by one of these agents.

Iodine labelled fatty acids

The topic of metabolic imaging is being covered elsewhere in this issue. It has been hoped that iodine labelled fatty acids would not only provide a marker of myocardial perfusion but also of the integrity of the metabolic pathways as fatty acids are a significant myocardial metabolic substrate. The issue of iodine uptake and washout has remained contentious however, and it is not really clear as yet what information is available from clearance times from the myocardium.[9]

SINGLE PHOTON EMISSION COMPUTERIZED TOMOGRAPHY (SPECT)

SPECT is being used with increasing frequency in nuclear medicine but only recently has the instrumentation been available from most of the major suppliers of nuclear medicine equipment for routine clinical use. SPECT has evolved to produce an image of tracer distribution within an organ as a 3 dimensional display and is usually performed with rotating gamma cameras.[10] SPECT has evolved because conventional planar imaging has the disadvantage that all information from a 3 dimensional organ is displayed as a 2 dimensional image; there is thus no information on different tracer uptake at different depths within the organ. Besides acquiring 3 dimensional imaging SPECT can eliminate activity which is superimposed upon the organ of interest and may degrade the image. SPECT has been used for thallium perfusion imaging, myocardial infarct imaging using ^{99m}Tc pyrophosphate infarct imaging and for gated blood pool imaging using labelled red cells.[3,11]

POSITRON EMISSION TOMOGRAPHY (PET)

A positron is a high energy positive electron emitted from certain radio isotopes which are generally produced from a cyclotron and have a very short half-life. The 1022 keV positive electron decays in what is known as an annihilation reaction with the production of two gamma emissions of 511 keV each which have the unique property of travelling at exactly 180° to each other. By assembling an array of detectors around the emitting source, images of very high resolution can be obtained as the only events that are regarded as valid are those that occur when a pair of both photons travelling away from each other at 180° strike a pair of detectors simultaneously. Photons which are slightly scattered will not strike the diametrically opposed detectors at the same time and will thus be rejected as invalid events by anti-coincidence logic. Positron imaging agents such as carbon-11 can be tagged to agents such as palmitic acid, fluorine-18 can be labelled to deoxyglucose and nitrogen-13 can be labelled to glutamic acid. In this way fatty acid, glucose, and amino acid metabolism in the heart can be studied.[12,13] Because the agents have a rapid half-life they are usually administered by continuous infusion before and during an intervention. Thus moment to moment changes in the way the heart is behaving under, for example pacing induced ischaemia, can be assessed. It is evident that positron cameras and the accompanying computers are extremely expensive and beyond the scope of most clinical nuclear cardiology departments. In addition one is dependent upon a fully functioning cyclotron on site.

BLOOD POOL STUDIES

The left and right ventricles may be imaged by either first pass or equilibrium gated techniques. The first pass method quite simply involves the injection of technetium-99m either as unbound pertechnetate or possibly labelled to the patient's own red cells.

The dose of technetium must be prepared with high specific activity, i.e. contained in a small volume and injected as a bolus usually into a peripheral vein with a rapid saline flush. Imaging is only carried out as the bolus passes through the central circulation once. Thus imaging takes only 30 seconds. The equilibrium gated technique involves the labelling of the entire blood pool usually by tagging the patients own red cells with technetium prior to imaging being carried out. Imaging is commenced once equilibration of the labelled red cells has taken place within the blood pool, and takes several minutes. In order for the first pass technique to be accurate a gamma camera with high count rate capabilities must be used in order to register enough photons during the first pass phase to produce statistically reliable images. A multicrystal camera (system 77, Baird Corporation) or the newer Scinticor (Scinticor Inc.) is able to meet these criteria more readily than single crystal cameras, although some of the newer digital single crystal cameras can produce perfectly adequate first pass images. Detection of end diastole and end systole is done directly from the time activity curve from the left ventricular region of interest, as each beat of the first pass phase is represented as a peak and a trough. The reader is referred elsewhere for more detailed description.[14] The equilibrium gated technique has really evolved because of the problem of adequate count rates as described above. In order to produce statistically reliable images, several hundred cardiac cycles need to be summed by the computer. Time resolution is carried out using the ECG gating system, whereby corresponding time slices from individual cardiac cycles are summed together. In this way, for example, the first 40 milliseconds of data from beat 1 is added to the first 40 milliseconds of beat 2 etc, and the sequence repeated for the second 40 milliseconds of beat 1 and 2 etc. A representative cycle from corresponding time slices of several hundred cardiac cycles can then be displayed. The equilibrium gated technique can therefore be used by any nuclear medicine department that has a reasonably modern gamma camera and the computing power for simple gating.

Both first pass and equilibrium gated techniques have advantages and disadvantages which are too detailed to go into in this article and the reader is referred elsewhere.[5,14] In addition to the images numerical data such as ejection fraction and cardiac volumes may be obtained from these scans and provided the temporal resolution of the time activity curves is adequate, emptying and filling rates may also be obtained.

THE NON IMAGING NUCLEAR PROBE

This is a device for measuring cardiac function by recording emitted radiation from the left ventricle following blood pool labelling with technetium in the same way as is carried out with an equilibrium blood pool scan. The devices are small and mobile and are cheaper to buy than conventional gamma cameras. Their main advantage is their extremely high sensitivity and they consist basically of a sodium iodide crystal with a single hole converging collimator mounted on a flexible arm, rather like an angle poise lamp. The high sensitivity enables sampling to be carried out at 10 msec intervals and therefore high temporal resolution beat to beat studies can be acquired. Using ECG gating representative time activity curves, similar to those produced in the equilibrium imaging technique can be produced. The disadvantage is that there is no visual display or image and one can never be totally certain of the positioning of the probe. The term 'nuclear stethoscope' has been coined to describe this piece of equipment and its validation and uses are described elsewhere.[15] It is not really useful as a diagnostic device.

REFERENCES

1 Elmaleh DR, van der Wall EE, Livni E, Miller BD, Strauss HW. Radiopharmaceuticals for cardiovascular nuclear medicine. In: van der Wall EE ed Non-invasive imaging of cardiac metabolism. Dordrecht: Martinus Nijhoff, 1987: pp. 1–37
2 Parkey RW, Bonte FJ, Meyer SL et al. A new method for radionuclide imaging of acute myocardial infarction in humans. Circulation 1974; 50: 540–546
3 Holman BL, Goldhaber SZ, Kirsch CM et al. Measurement of infarct size using single photon emission computed tomography and technetium-99m pyrophosphate: a description of the method and comparison with patient prognosis. Am J Cardiol 1982; 50: 503–511
4 Addonizio LJ, Michler RE, Marboe C et al. Imaging of cardiac allograft rejection in dogs using indium-111 monoclonal antimyosin Fab. J Am Coll Cardiol 1987; 9: 555–564
5 Dymond DS. Standards for acquisition, data analysis and interpretation of myocardial scintigraphy and blood pool scintigraphy. In: Simoons ML, Reiber JHC eds. Nuclear Imaging in Clinical Cardiology, Boston: Martinus Nijhoff, 1984: pp. 233–252
6 Maddahi J, Garcia EV, Berman DS. Quantitative analysis of the distribution and washout of thallium-201 in the myocardium: description of the method and its clinical application. In: Simoons ML, Reiber JHC eds. Nuclear Imaging in Clinical Cardiology. Boston: Martinus Nijhoff, 1984: 103–124
7 Gibson RS, Watson DD, Carabello BA, Holt ND, Bellar GA. Clinical implications of increased lung uptake of thallium-201 during exercise scintigraphy two weeks after myocardial infarction. Am J Cardiol 1982; 49: 1586–1593
8 Kiat H, Maddahi J, Roy LT et al. Comparison of Technetium-99m MIBI and

thallium-201 for evaluation of coronary artery disease by planar and tomographic methods. Am Heart J 1989; 117: 1–11

9 Visser FC, Westera G. Radio-iodinated free fatty acids: a clue to myocardial metabolism? In: van der Wall EE ed. Non-invasive imaging of cardiac metabolism. Dordrecht: Martinus Nijhoff, 1987: pp. 127–138

10 Coleman RE, Blinder RA, Jaszczak RJ. Single photon emission computed tomography (SPECT). part 2: clinical applications. Invest Radiol 1986; 21: 1–11

11 Corbett JR, Jansen DE, Lewis SE et al. Tomographic gated blood pool radionuclide ventriculography: analysis of wall motion and left ventricular volumes in patients with coronary artery disease. J Am Coll Cardiol 1985; 6: 349–358

12 Fox KAA, Knabb RM, Bergmann SR, Sobel BE. Progress in cardiac positron emission tomography with emphasis on carbon-11 labelled palmitate and oxygen-15 labelled water. In: van der Wall EE ed. Non-invasive imaging of cardiac metabolism. Dordrecht: Martinus Nijhoff, Dordrecht 1987: pp. 203–240

13 Landsheere CM. Assessment of glucose utilisation in normal and ischaemic myocardium with positron emission tomography and 18 F-deoxyglucose. In: van der Wall EE ed. Non-invasive imaging of cardiac metabolism. Dordrecht: Martinus Nijhoff, 1987: pp. 241–263

14 Zaret BL, Berger HJ. First-pass and equilibrium radionuclide angiocardiography for evaluating ventricular performance. In: Simoons ML, Reiber JHC eds. Nuclear Imaging in Clinical Cardiology, Boston: Martinus Nijhoff, 1984: pp. 125–151

15 Berger HJ, Davies RA, Batsford WP, Hoffer PB, Gottschalf A, Zaret BL. Beat to beat left ventricular performance assessed from the equilbrium cardiac blood pool using a computerised nuclear probe. Circulation 1981; 63: 133–142

British Medical Bulletin (1989) Vol. 45, No. 4, pp. 848–880
© The British Council 1989

The principles of magnetic resonance

D B Longmore
Magnetic Resonance Unit, The National Heart and Chest Hospitals, London, UK

Magnetic Resonance (MR), which has no known biological hazard, is capable of producing high resolution thin tomographic images in any plane and blocks of 3-dimensional information. It can be used to study blood flow and to gain information about the composition of important materials seen and quantified on dimensionally accurate images.

The MR image is a thin tomographic slice or a true three dimensional block of data which can be reconstructed in any desired way rather than a shadowgram of all the structures in the beam. It is the only imaging technique which can acquire data in a 3-dimensional format. CT images can be reconstructed to form a pseudo 3-D image or a hologram but the flexibility conferred by acquiring the data as a true 3-D block gives many advantages.

The spatial resolution of MR images are theoretically those of low powered microscopy, the practical limits with the present generation of equipment are voxel sizes of one third by one third by two millimetres.

The term Magnetic Resonance Imaging (MRI) is used commonly, particularly in the USA, avoiding association with the term, nuclear, and emphasizing the imaging potential of the technique. The terms Nuclear Magnetic Resonance (NMR) or Magnetic Resonance (MR) more correctly describe the most powerful diagnostic instrument yet devised. The simplified description of the phenomena involved in MR which follows is intended to be comprehensive and does not require foreknowledge of classical physics, quantum mechanics, fluency with mathematical formulae or an understanding of image reconstruction.

There are many explanations of MR, some omitting the

0007–1420/89/0045–0848/$10.00

more difficult concepts. An accurate, comprehensive description is found on the textbook on MR by Gadian, *Nuclear Magnetic Resonance and its Applicatons for Living Systems* (Oxford University Press, 1982).

The phenomenon of Nuclear Magnetic Resonance was discovered in 1946 by two Americans, Bloch and Purcell. They were jointly awarded a Nobel Prize. The basic physics and many of the facts described in the section on how MR works are even older. Democrates, a Greek philosopher in the 5th Century BC described what was until recently thought to be the smallest indivisible particle of matter, the atom (Greek atomos-indivisible). In the 1st Century BC, the Roman philosopher, Lucretius, described atoms as hard, solid objects moving at great speeds, colliding and sticking in combination.

The first of the many theories of the new physics about the structure of the atom relevant to the discovery of NMR are also old. Early significant theories are the quantum theory (Max Planck 1900) and the theory of relativity (Albert Einstein 1905).

The mathematics on which image reconstruction is based were defined by Fourier, a Frenchman, who was a friend of Napoleon. The relationship between the frequency of precession and field strength was described by Joseph Larmor, an Irish physicist, at the turn of the century. NMR has been used as a routine method of chemical analysis for nearly 30 years.

It was a logical extension of its application in the analytical chemistry laboratory to attempt to use NMR to give an insight into metabolic processes. The clinical application of spectroscopy was pioneered by George Radda in Oxford. (There are no practical applications of spectroscopy in the chest and Magnetic Resonance Spectroscopy (MRS) is not discussed in this chapter.)

In 1973, Paul Lauterbur in the USA wrote a paper in Nature explaining how the NMR signal might be used to produce an image, followed by a paper from Richard Ernst in Switzerland, who described a different method. Shortly after, Hinshaw and Moore of Nottingham University, described a further ingenious way of producing an image from an NMR signal.

In 1976, using a rapid imaging technique which will eventually come into routine use, Professor Peter Mansfield, also at Nottingham, produced the first human image.

By this time, Damadian, in the United States, had performed the remarkable feat of designing and building a superconducting magnet and all the hardware and software for a whole body imager. In Aberdeen, Hutchinson and others were working on a cheaper method of producing an imager but *M and D*, the company formed to develop these ideas, was underfunded and failed.

Using yet another technique, Hounsfield and his co-workers, including Young at EMI Medical, produced the first commercial whole body imager which has been in use at the Hammersmith Hospital for 9 years. The superconducting magnet for the EMI machine was made at *Oxford Instruments*, who soon became the supplier of over 90% of the world's superconducting magnets.

ESSENTIALS OF MR

This section is designed to contain enough information to understand the basic principles of MR. It deals with the basic physics, the production of the MR signal and the creation of an image from the MR signal.

It is difficult to describe the mechanism of the generation of the NMR signal without resorting to mathematical descriptions. The problem which besets all who try is the inter-relationship between classical physics, which is logical and easy to comprehend, on the one hand, and on the other hand, quantum mechanics, relativity and the interaction between the four forces of nature. These are more complex and, possibly because they are not fully understood, cannot readily be described in normal logical terms. This description is designed to be complementary to the series of diagrams which accompany it. It is suggested that the reader understands one section at a time, the subject divides naturally into three sections—production of the NMR signal, scanning technique, and image reconstruction. Only the first of these is difficult for the reasons given above.

This section contains a series of diagrams with captions which should be studied after reading the description given below. The description omits some aspects of MR which are best dealt with diagrammatically whilst the diagrams, for the sake of brevity, are not totally comprehensive. Both are needed for a full understanding.

Structure of an atom

Most of the energy and matter in the universe is concentrated in the stars and the suns which are at such high temperatures that matter exists as an amorphous plasma consisting of charged particles moving at great speeds and without structure. In the cooler parts of the universe such as the earth, the fundamental particles and packets of energy are organized into sub-atomic structures which in turn come together to form atoms.

At temperatures above absolute zero, atoms are not static structures but are a turmoil of activity. The anatomy of an atom is not known in detail because there is no known method of visualizing it. At the moment, the only way of finding out about the contents of an atom and particularly its nucleus, is to bombard it with particles which are accelerated to speeds approaching the speed of light so that they contain enormous energies and to see what smaller particles can be produced. It is not known whether these smaller particles actually existed in the intact nucleus or whether they were created by the bombardment. Experiments of this kind combined with mathematical studies of the charges, the forces, the masses and the angular rotation of the building bricks of the nucleus, appear to reveal a complicated inter-relationship between hundreds of particles of known weight, weightless particles, packets of energy, with and without mass, all of which have effects on each other, some exhibiting strong or weak attracting forces on their neighbours and others carrying fractions of an electric charge. Many particles or energies appear to co-exist with corresponding anti-particles or opposite energies.

Whatever the basic components of a nucleus might be, the overall effect is a positively charged mass of matter and energy. Related to the nucleus, but at relatively great distances from it, are negatively charged electrons travelling at nearly the speed of light. These electrons are statistically more likely to be in a particular area related to the nucleus and are joined to it by eletromagnetic forces which exert some effects on the nucleus relevant to NMR behaviour.

Hydrogen atom

The hydrogen atom is the simplest atom. Its nucleus, termed the proton, contains a single positive charge and it has one negatively charged electron related to it. Hydrogen is the most common element in the universe and is present in body water, making up 70% of our body weight, and in most organic materials. It is therefore abundant in the body and all the studies described in this chapter are of the proton (Fig.1).

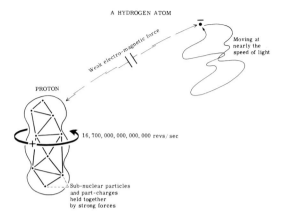

Fig. 1 Hydrogen is the most abundant material in the universe. Its atom is the simplest with a single positively charged nuclear particle termed a proton and a single much lighter negatively charged electron loosely bound to it by electromagnetic forces. The electron is more likely to be found in a particular region at a great distance from the nucleus, although it can be anywhere, even associated with a nucleus. The proton in turn consists of many smaller sub-atomic particles, packets (quanta) of energy and various forces. The proton spins on its long axis about one billion billion (10^{24}) times per minute or 1.66×10^{22} cycles per second (Hz).

Nuclear spin

The proton spins on its axis at about a billion billion 10^{24} revolutions per minute or 16 billion per second (1.66×10^{22} Hz). The proton is small and the speed of its surface is therefore less than the speed of light. Some larger and heavier atoms containing an even number of protons do not exhibit the properties of spin. A simplified explanation is that because pairs of protons spin in opposite directions, cancelling out the effect. Other structures found in the nucleus (nucleons) include neutrons, which appear to be identical with the proton except that they carry an electron in combination. The neutrons also spin and if there is an even number of neutrons and protons, there is no overall spin because of the cancellation effect. Only certain atoms with an odd number of nucleons (protons and neutrons) exhibit net spin (Figs.2, 3).

Magnetism

Several kinds of magnetism exist related to atomic structure; in this chapter only nuclear magnetism is considered. The familiar ferromagnetism and nuclear magnetism are relevant.

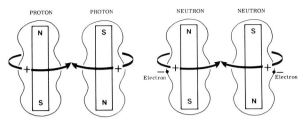

Fig. 2 When protons and neutrons exist together in pairs, their magnetic dipoles are orientated opposite each other. The spin of one proton opposes the spin of another proton, therefore there is no net spin. Similarly, the spin of a neutron can be opposed by that of another neutron, again producing no net spin. But the spin of a neutron cannot cancel that of a proton. There is only net spin and therefore a magnetic field when there is an odd number of protons or neutrons.

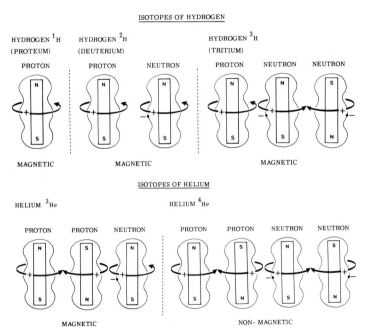

Fig. 3 All of the 280 stable atomic nuclei consist of protons and neutrons. Approximately 100 of them are magnetic because they contain unpaired protons or neutrons. The five simplest nuclei are used to illustrate this point.

Nuclear magnetism

Spinning nuclei carrying a positive electric charge behave like an electric current passing around a loop and generate a magnetic field. The spinning nuclei therefore behave like very weak, tiny bar magnets (Fig.4).

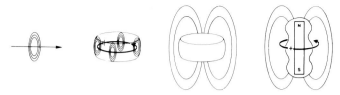

Fig. 4 (From left to right) A magnetic field around a wire carrying an electric current. A ring of wire carrying a current (a current loop) generating a symmetrical magnetic field. Typical lines of magnetic force generated by a current loop. The rotating positive charge on the spinning proton behaves like a current loop generating a magnetic field.

Each nuclear magnet (for the purpose of this description each proton) is surrounded by a magnetic field and behaves like a small bar magnet. They align themselves like compass needles in a magnetic field. There are two unusual features about this alignment: nuclear alignment and nuclear precession.

Nuclear alignment

Unlike compass needles which will always align with the north seeking pole pointing north and the south seeking pole pointing south, atomic nuclei align in almost equal numbers with the north seeking pole pointing north and with the north seeking pole pointing south. The numbers are not quite equal. The ratio of high energy to low energy protons increases proportionally with field strength. At a field strength of 0.5 Tesla, about six in every million nuclei more point in the expected direction than the unexpected direction. The nuclei which are pointing in the correct direction (north seeking pointing north are said to be in a lower energy state than those which are 'the wrong way round', with the north seeking pole pointing south, which are said to be in a high energy state. The application of a suitable energy source to the system can change the ratio of the high and low energy states, putting more nuclei into the high energy state (Fig.5).

Nuclear precession

At all temperatures above absolute zero, under the influence of thermal energy, the spinning nuclei do not remain aligned with the lines of force in a magnetic field. They are perturbed and instead of spinning on an axis exactly in line with an external magnetic field, they are pushed to one side and wobble about the axis in a

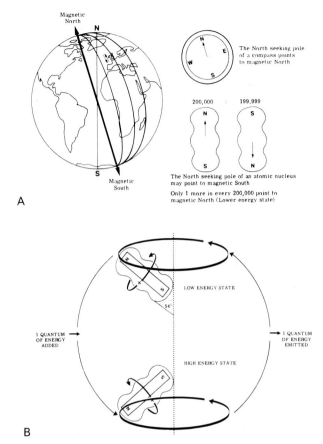

Fig. 5 Energy states **A.** Unlike compass needles which only align with the north seeking pole seeking north, magnetic nuclei align themselves in one of two ways: (1) the north seeking pole seeking north (parallel); (2) The north seeking pole seeking south (anti-parallel). The north seeking nucleus is said to be in a lower energy state and the south seeking nucleus in a higher energy state. There are only two allowed states because the higher energy state contains one minimum unit of energy (a quantum) more than the nucleus in the lower energy state. Only 1 more nucleus in every 200,000 is in the lower energy state. **B.** Shows the precessing proton in the 2 possible energy states separated by one quantum of energy.

similar way to a spinning top which has been pushed away from the vertical. This motion is known as precession (Fig.6).

Resonance frequency (Larmor frequency)

The rate of precession is much lower than the rate of spin. A spinning top rotating at about a thousand rpm will precess at a few

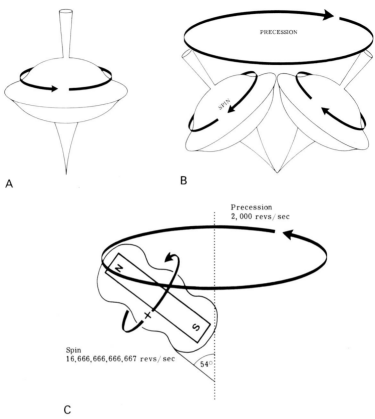

Fig. 6 The concept of precession. A spinning object which is deflected to one side in a magnetic field 'precesses' at a much slower rate than its rate of spin. A proton spinning at one billion billion rpm precesses at a rate of approximately 2 kHz in the earth's magnetic field. **A.** Shows a spinning top in the earth's gravitational field. **B.** Shows the same top deflected to one side 'precessing' about its axis at a slower rate than its spin. **C.** Illustrates hydrogen proton spin in a 0.5 Gauss magnetic field. Quantum mechanics dictates that the angle of precession is 54 degrees.

rpm. The atomic nuclei spinning at about a billion billion rpm precess much more slowly at a frequency related to the strength of the background magnetic field. Protons in the earth's field precess at a few kilohertz. At 0.25 Tesla (1 Tesla = 10,000 Gauss, 1 Gauss = about 1.75 of the earth's magnetic field), the precession rate is 14 MHz. In a commonly used imaging field strength of 0.5 Tesla approaching 10,000 times the earth's magnetic field, the proton precesses at about 21 MHz (Fig.7).

This relationship between the frequency of precession and the

PRECESSIONAL FREQUENCIES

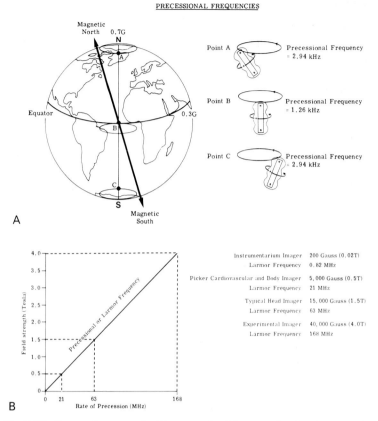

Fig. 7 The Larmor frequency. **A.** The precessional frequency is related to magnetic field strength. Precessional frequency is greater in a stronger field. Examples of the precessional frequency of hydrogen protons in water in the earth's magnetic field, which is stronger at the poles, 0.7 Gauss (Points A and C) than it is at the equator, 0.3 Gauss (Point B), are shown. The relationship between field strength and precessional frequency for hydrogen protons in water is 4.2 kHz/Gauss or 42 MHz/Tesla. Therefore hydrogen protons in water, and in us, precess at 2.94 kHz at the poles and at 1.26 kHz at the equator. **B.** Shows the Larmor frequency for typical imagers, and research machines.

magnetic field strength is known as the Larmor frequency or the resonant frequency. This relationship is the key to nuclear magnetic resonance imaging.

Nuclei of different elements have different magnetization and have a different Larmor frequency in the same magnetic field. For example, the phosphorus nucleus precesses at a slower speed than the proton at about 9 MHz in an 0.5 Tesla field.

Quantum effects

This description of magnetic resonance has been based on classical physics. However, many of the phenomena described do not fit the rules of classical physics and need to be described in terms of quantum physics.

Energy is only available in certain units known as quanta. While a spinning top is being pushed to one side, it appears to precess through an infinite number of angles. In fact, it moves through a very large number of extremely small discrete steps because the energy available to push it to one side comes in finite, tiny packages—quanta. The quanta of energy are minute compared with the size of the system in the example of the spinning top. The nuclear mass, however, is very small and a quantum of energy pushes it a finite distance. One or more quanta will suffice to push a proton from a low energy state to a high energy state.

Just as the two allowed states of parallel and anti-parallel are dictated by quantum physics, so is the angle of precession. For the proton, this angle is fixed at 54 degrees. Therefore, in a magnetic field in a typical imager with a magnetic field strength of 0.5 Tesla, the protons will be precessing aligned along the length of the lines of force with 200,000 protons in the high energy state lying 'the wrong way round' to every 200,001 lying in the low energy state the 'right way round'. The protons which are spinning on their axes at 10^{22} revolutions a minute will be precessing about an angle of 54 degrees at 21×10^6 cycles a second.

Net magnetism

So far, this description has only dealt with individual protons precessing in the high and low energy states. From this stage onwards, this description will deal with the net effects or 'crowd behaviour' of countless billions of protons (Fig.8).

The overall effect of the protons aligned and precessing along the lines of force of the applied field is a weak magnetic field generated by the excess of protons in the low energy state, lying parallel over high energy protons lying anti-parallel. If all the protons within us were aligned in the expected low energy state or in the opposite direction, we would be 200,000 times as magnetic and could not move freely in the earth's field.

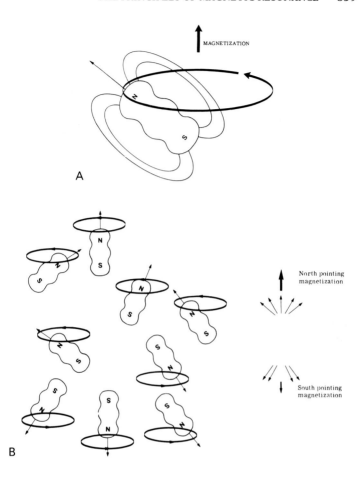

MAGNETIZATION

A

North pointing
magnetization

South pointing
magnetization

B

NET MAGNETIZATION

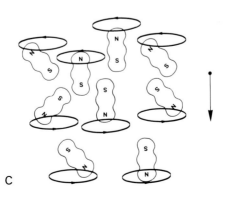

C

Axis of magnetization

The long axis of the magnetic field inside a solenoid magnet is conventionally known as the z axis. The parallel lines of force of the field between the poles of a permanent or yoke-shaped electromagnet are also said to be in the z axis. The plane horizontally across the magnet is conventionally described as the x axis and vertically as the y axis. Thus, in the resting state, the magnetic force generated by the protons lying along the lines of force of the magnet are said to be generating a field in the z axis.

It is conventional to describe the net axis of magnetization as if it can exist in any plane related to the x, y and z axes. Indeed, the magnetization can exist in any plane but, in fact, angles different from the z axis only exist because of a difference in the ratio between protons in the high energy state and the low energy state.

Rotating frame of reference

To make the descriptions of the effects of radio pulses and an understanding of the signals generated, it is usual to view the MR system as if the observer is rotating at the Larmor frequency. In the case of a 0.5 T machine, it is as if the observer is rotating round the patient 21 million times a second. This convention simplifies diagrammatic representations of the phenomena. In some diagrams, a small arrow represents the imaginary movement of the observer in the rotating frame of reference. This convention is particularly useful when considering phenomena like T2 relaxation and phase shift discussed below.

Relationship between nuclear precession and radio frequency

A sensitive radio receiver with its aerial placed near any material at a temperature above absolute zero will detect a faint hiss of radio

---

Fig. 8 A. Each proton has a tiny magnetic field surrounding its long axis which has both magnitude and direction as shown by the vector arrow. As this vector is constantly moving, due to precession, the net magnetic vector of the single proton along the axis of precession is shown by the closed arrow. **B.** The overall effect of countless billions of magnetic vectors is to produce an overall net magnetization vector. 5 protons are shown in the low energy state with their magnetic vectors pointing north, or parallel, which is stronger than magnetic vectors of the 4 protons in the high energy state with their magnetic vectors pointing south, or anti-parallel. **C.** Illustrates that if the excess of protons are in the high energy state, then the overall net magnetization is displaced through 180 degrees and points south or anti-parallel.

RELATIONSHIP BETWEEN PRECESSION AND ELECTROMAGNETIC INDUCTION

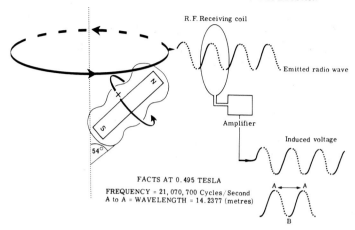

Fig. 9 Relationship between precession and electromagnetic induction. A moving magnetic field (the precessing proton) generates an electromagnetic wave which has the same frequency as the rate of precession of the proton (21 MHz in a 0.5 T imager). If a receiver aerial was to detect the emitted radio wave, the amplitude and frequency of the voltage induced in the aerial will be directly proportional to the amplitude and frequency of the radio wave and therefore the precessional rate and direction of the proton. A positive voltage is induced as the proton moves towards the receiver and a negative voltage induced as the proton moves away from the receiver as shown.

noise, known as Johnson noise. This is caused by moving charged particles including the net magnetization of nuclei precessing randomly. An aerial placed around a patient in the magnet would also detect a random hiss of radio noise due to the same cause (Fig.9).

If the protons in the patient or a region of the patient could be persuaded to precess in unison instead of in a random manner, the incoherent radio hiss would be converted to a cohesive signal. The net magnetization caused by the precessing nuclei rotating within the aerial would induce an alternating voltage in the aerial. The mechanism of this induction is the relationship between the electromagnetic force generated by the net magnetism of the precessing nuclei and the voltage induced in the aerial.

Two effects of energy applied at the resonant frequency

The magnetic resonance signal is generated by putting small amounts of energy into the system to bring about this cohesion. The energy is applied using radio-frequency energy transmitted through aerials near to the patient. The radio-frequency energy will only couple with and influence the precession of nuclei only if the frequency corresponds with the Larmor or resonant frequency. If radio-frequency energy is applied at other frequencies, it has no effect. The energy applied at the Larmor frequency has two effects.

Moving nuclei from the low energy state to the high energy state

Energy applied at the resonant Larmor frequency will cause some nuclei to move from the low energy state to the high energy state (Fig.10).

Putting the nuclei into phase

Normally the protons are precessing in the two energy states randomly. The RF pulse at the Larmor frequency has the effect of gathering the precessing protons and making them precess together (in phase). This process sometimes known as requantising takes place so quickly that the effect can be regarded as instantaneous. The magnetic component of the RF pulse is very small in comparison to the main field and it is remarkable that this weak

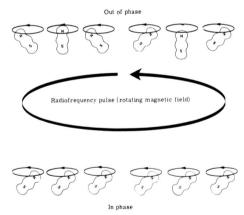

Fig. 10 When energy in the form of a radiofrequency (RF) pulse at the Larmor frequency is added to the system, two phenomena occur. Firstly, the ratio of parallel to anti-parallel protons is altered and, secondly, the protons which were all precessing randomly precess in unison. This can simply be explained by considering the RF pulse as a rotating magnetic field. As all the protons experience the same force or 'push' at the same time, eventually they will all precess in unison or 'in phase'. This effect takes place so rapidly that it can be regarded as instantaneous.

rotating field at a strength of a few microtesla at the resonant frequency can influence protons in a field of up to several Tesla many millions as strong (Figs.11–12).

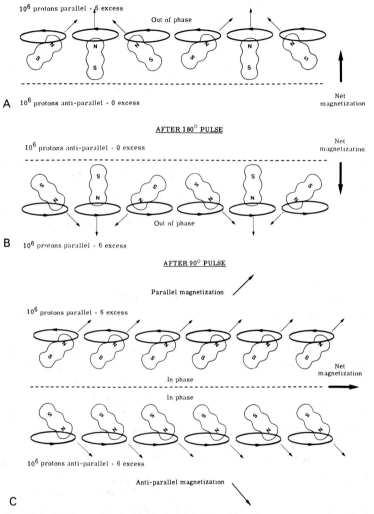

Fig. 11 A. In the equilibrium state in a 0.5 T machine, there are approximately 6 excess protons in the low energy state with a resultant parallel net magnetization. **B.** After a 180 degree pulse, the 6 excess are in the high energy state with the net magnetization displaced through 180 degrees into the anti-parallel direction. **C.** After a 90 degree pulse the number of protons parallel and anti-parallel are equal, with the resultant net magnetization displaced into the xy plane mid-way between parallel and anti-parallel; i.e. the xy plane. Also note that the protons are now precessing 'in phase.'

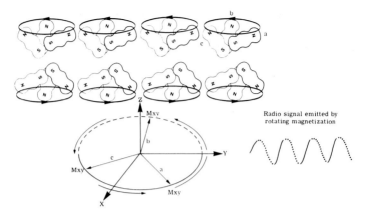

Fig. 12 Protons precessing 'in-phase'. The net magnetization rotates in the xy plane after a 90 degree pulse. This is due to the parallel and anti-parallel protons precessing in phase. When the protons are at position (a) around their precessional motion the direction of the net magnetization in the xy plane is shown. As the protons precess to position (b), the net magnetization also rotates as indicated, and so on to position (c). The effect is that of a rotating net magnetization.

Relaxation times T1 (Spin lattice relaxation)

After energy has been applied to change the net magnetization vector from the resting low energy state where it is in line with the magnetic field to the high energy state where it may lie in the opposite direction, nuclei move back one at a time to the original resting state. They do so at a steady rate producing an exponential recovery of the original net magnetization in the z axis from the opposite direction (the z axis). The time taken for this relaxation to take place for the protons in pure water is several seconds. In body fluids and in cellular water it is more typically one second or less. This time is known as T1. It is actually the time taken for 63% of the protons to return to the normal resting position (Fig.13).

The energy which was applied in the RF pulse is lost as heat into the molecular lattice of the patient and T1 relaxation is sometimes known as spin lattice relaxation. At the half way stage, the magnetization vector is not parallel to the field in the low energy state or anti-parallel to it in the high energy state, but is rotating around the axis at the Larmor frequency. This phenomenon is discussed in more detail below under the head of 'Pulse Angle'.

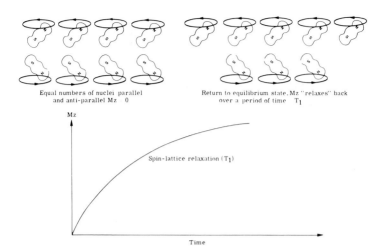

Equal numbers of nuclei parallel and anti-parallel Mz 0

Return to equilibrium state, Mz "relaxes" back over a period of time T_1

Mz

Spin-lattice relaxation (T_1)

Time

Fig. 13 Spin Lattice relaxation–T1. After RF energy has been added to the system displacing the net magnetization, nuclei move back from their high energy state to the low energy state one at a time, at a steady rate producing an exponential recovery back to the equilibrium state. The energy lost by each proton is in the form of a quantum of heat to its surrounding molecular lattice and is therefore termed Spin Lattice Relaxation or T1. For mathematical reasons T1 is taken to be the time for 63% of the protons to revert back to their original low energy state.

T2 Relaxation (Spin spin relaxation)

When the protons are spinning cohesively in phase and the net magnetization is in the xy plane, a voltage at the resonant frequency is induced in a detector aerial placed around the patient. This voltage which diminishes rapidly is known as the free induction decay. The loss of signal is due to two factors.

Protons precess at a rate related to their local magnetic field. Protons in some chemical environments precess more rapidly, for example the protons precessing in pure water at 0.5 Tesla precess at a frequency of 70 Hz faster than in fat. Very few areas in the body are made up of pure chemicals and the protons all experience different local magnetic fields.

The exponential loss of signal due to differences in local magnetic field is known as T2. The loss of signal due to T2 is sometimes known as spin spin relaxation because it is due to local molecular effects. T2 is always shorter than T1. In biological systems, T2 is usually less than 40 msecs (Fig.14).

The magnet creating the field in which the patient lies may not

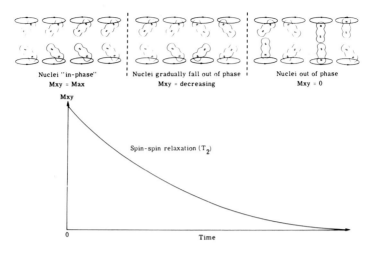

Nuclei "in-phase"   Nuclei gradually fall out of phase   Nuclei out of phase
Mxy = Max   Mxy = decreasing   Mxy = 0

Spin-spin relaxation (T_2)

Fig. 14 Spin Spin relaxation–T2. When RF energy is added to the system, the protons precess in phase. The rate of precession, as previously described, is related to the local magnetic field strength (Larmor Principle). Individual protons, in vivo, will all experience differing magnetic fields depending on the local chemical environment. Some protons may be close to strongly magnetic atoms or molecules, such as ferromagnetic atoms like iron and others close to weakly magnetic atoms. The result of protons experiencing differing magnetic environments is that the precessional frequencies will vary from proton to proton. They therefore cease to precess in phase and will eventually precess, as in the equilibrium state, completely out of phase, and no signal will be detected. The time taken for this loss of phase is termed Spin Spin Relaxation or T2.

produce a perfectly homogenous field. It is very difficult to produce a large volume inside a magnet in which the magnetic field strength is perfectly uniform. Inhomogeneity of the magnet means that some parts of the patient are in a higher field of strength than others, therefore the precessional frequencies will vary. Even if a magnet is virtually perfect, the presence of a patient within it consisting of various weakly magnetic materials and containing iron will distort the field and some protons will be in a slightly stronger magnetic field than others. The combined exponential loss of signal due to field inhomogeneity and T2 are usually considered together under the heading T2* (Fig.15).

A large effort has been devoted to using T1 and T2 measurements to define pathological processes. It takes a long time to obtain a complete and accurate T1 or T2 measurement and most of the work which has been done is empirical and not very convincing. It does appear, however, that malignant tumours in

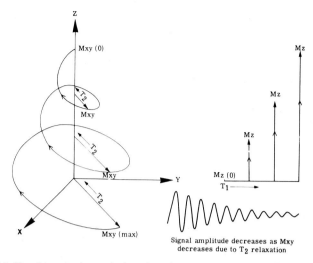

Fig. 15 Signal is only detected when there is an xy component to the rotating net magnetization. Because of T1 and T2* effects net magnetization in the xy plane decreases exponentially. The resultant detectable signal therefore decays in the same manner and is known as the free induction decay (FID).

the chest have prolonged T1 and T2. A compromise instead of measuring T1 and T2 properly is to use a sequence which emphasizes one or the other. It is fashionable to refer to T1-weighted and T2-weighted images. It must be remembered, however, that the images are in fact proton density maps usually with a slight emphasis towards T1 or T2. They have been likened to a roast beef dinner with pepper or salt added. In the section on sequences below, the method of obtaining T1 or T2 weighting is described.

Pulse angle (Flip angle, inversion)

Transition of protons from the low energy state to the high energy state changes the net effect of their magnetism. In the natural state with the patient lying in a magnetic field (the earth's magnetic field or a much more powerful field created by a magnet), the net magnetization caused by the small excess of protons in the low energy state over those in the high energy state is in the direction of the field. The radio energy applied to the system has the two effects of putting the protons into phase and influencing the number of protons moving from the low energy state to the high energy state and thus the net magnetism. The amount of radio energy causing the change of energy state is related to the power of the transmitter at the Larmor frequency and the duration of the applied RF at the frequency. A high powered transmitter putting energy into the system in a short pulse is more efficient than a lower powered transmitter over a longer transmission period. During the stimulation, protons are relaxing to the resting state and dephasing. The individual nuclei pass from the low to the high energy state instantaneously but the net effect is as if the axis of magnetization is spiralling down at a rate proportional to the power of the RF pulse.

The application of the correct amount of RF energy will produce a 180 degree pulse with the net magnetization lying in the opposite direction to the natural state and producing no signal. Maximum signal can be produced by applying sufficient RF energy to achieve a 90 degree pulse with the net magnetization in the xy plane. This magnetization is lost quickly due to the T2* effects. The T2* effects can be cancelled after the signal has been lost by applying a 180 degree pulse so that the protons are now spinning in the opposite direction. The forces which were dephasing them now push them back into phase so that the signal which was lost is recaptured only to be lost again due to dephasing in the opposite direction when it can be recovered with the application of a further 180 degree pulse. The signal which is recaptured is known as a spin echo. A number of echoes can be recaptured in this way, each echo is slightly smaller than the previous echo because of the T1 effects.

What happens during a scan

This section relates the physics described above to a patient undergoing a magnetic resonance examination and deals with data acquisition and image reconstruction.

Within a few seconds of the patient being placed in the magnetic field, the nuclei will align and precess with their axes parallel to the main field in the high and low energy states with the magnetization vector along the long axis of the magnet producing no coherent radio signal.

In order to create an image, energy has to be put into a selected part of the patient to create an NMR signal. Several steps are necessary to encode the source of the signal in some way that will allow spatial resolution to be obtained for image construction.

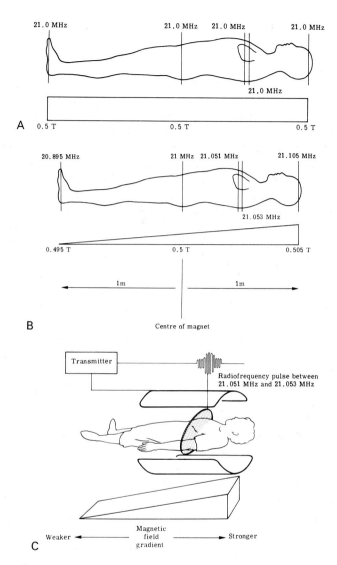

Fig. 16 Slice selection. **A.** If a subject is placed in a uniform magnetic field of 0.5 Tesla, hydrogen protons at every point along the subject will precess at the same frequency, i.e. 21×10^6 Hz (21 MHz). **B.** If the magnetic field strength at the head end of the subject was slightly stronger than at the foot end by applying a small magnetic gradient from foot to head, then protons at different points along the length of the subject would precess at slightly different frequencies, those protons at the head end precessing faster than those at the foot end. A typical 0.5 T imager applies a magnetic gradient of 5 millitesla (mT) per metre in either direction from the centre of the magnet. Hydrogen protons at the foot end (1 m from centre) will now precess at 20.895 MHz and those at the head end (1 m from centre) at 21.105

Slice selection

When a magnetic gradient is applied along the length of the patient from the head to the feet, due to the Larmor frequency each part of the body will contain protons precessing at a different frequency. A radio frequency pulse can be tailored in shape and frequency to excite a thin slice of the patient. In the case of a longitudinal magnetic gradient, the slice will be transverse. For coronal or sagittal slices, the gradient is applied from side to side or front to back of the patient. Oblique slices are more complex and a combination of two or more gradients must be applied to produce a plane of uniform magnetism through the patient. Theoretically, the plane could be curved to follow a curved structure in the chest. For example, the plane could be tailored to follow the curve of the aorta. In pratice, a curved plane is not used and curved structures in the chest are visualized by using a number of slices which are then reconstructed using a post image processing computer. The thickness of the slice can be varied in two ways because it depends on the steepness of the gradient and the bandwidth of the RF pulse. A steep gradient changes the frequency of the precession more rapidly, thus a radiofrequency pulse of a fixed bandwidth will resonate with a thinner slice of the patient. Alternatively, a radiofrequency pulse of a narrow bandwidth will also resonate with a thinner slice. The radiofrequency pulse is applied with a particular shape (known as a sync function) which Fourier transforms into a square wave thus the edges of the slice are sharply defined and there is no contribution to the image from tissues adjacent to it which would degrade flow and other measurements.

Various slice thicknesses can be used, the commonest being 10 mm. Thinner slices are desirable because they reduce the partial volume effect of a structure which is less than 10 mm thick passing along or obliquely through the slice. The amount of signal obtained from a slice depends on the number of protons in the slice and is reduced to 20% in a 2 mm slice. The background noise, however, produced by radio emissions from the remainder of the patient, remains constant, therefore the signal to noise ratio becomes less favourable (Fig.16).

MHz. **C.** A pulse of radio waves of a given frequency range will only excite protons that are precessing within the same frequency range. Only the protons in the desired anatomical 'slice' will be excited by a radio-frequency pulse of the appropriate frequency range, all other protons remaining unaffected. A 'slice' through the level of the heart is illustrated.

Image reconstruction—The spatial encoding gradients

Once a slice has been selected and the tissues within it have been excited, a free induction decay signal at the Larmor frequency is received in an aerial close to the patient. This signal arises from all of the protons in the slice and there is no spatial resolution.

Spatial resolution can only be obtained by applying further magnetic gradients to make protons precess a different frequencies in different parts of the patient. These gradients can be applied in one of three ways. In R theta reconstruction angular gradients are used which are rotated round the patient in steps of one or two degrees. The method of constructing the image from Fourier transformed readings of each slice to produce a profile of the proton density along each line is similar to the back projection methods used in CT scanning. This technique was used in some of the early machines. Although it has certain advantages, notably insensitivity to movement, it is not as useful in the chest as xy reconstruction which is described in detail below. (One advantage of R theta reconstruction is the ability to construct the image continuously so that a scan may be terminated as soon as there is enough information or it is obvious that the patient has moved and corrupted the scan. A disadvantage is the inevitable central artefact.) Once the reader has understood xy reconstruction, the difference between this and echo planar (and other one-shot methods) imaging is small and will be explained at the end of the section.

XY reconstruction

The xy reconstruction technique uses two separate gradients perpendicular to each other and to the slice selection gradient to produce a two dimensional image rather than one gradient at different angles round the z axis as in the R theta reconstruction. These gradients are applied separately, the first is known as the phase-encoding gradient and the second as the read gradient. It is easier to understand the function of these gradients if they are considered in the reverse order.

Read gradient

The read gradient is applied during data acquisition. Because of the Larmor frequency it has the effect of causing a gradation of the frequency of the signal emanating from the protons across the

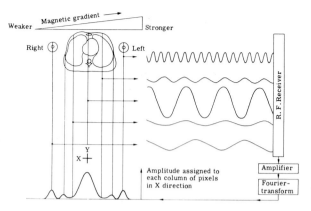

Fig. 17 Frequency Encoding. Signal is obtained from all hydrogen protons in the selected slice but contains no spatial information. A second magnetic gradient, the frequency encoding or 'read' gradient, is applied across the patient from right to left in the x direction. The amplitude of the signal will depend on the hydrogen proton density in the x direction. The frequency of the signals will depend on their position in the x direction. Signal from the stronger end of the gradient will have a higher frequency than that at the weaker end. The signal from the air filled lungs with relatively few hydrogen protons will have less amplitude than the signal obtained from the mediastinum which will contain many hydrogen protons. The mass of signals of different amplitudes and frequencies once amplified undergo fast Fourier Transformation. The result is that the correct amplitude is assigned to each frequency and therefore to each column of pixels in the x direction.

patient. A high frequency Fourier transformation applied to the jumble of radio signal consisting of mixed frequencies produces a spectrum of frequency and power. The frequency relates to the position and the power to the number of protons. Although the transformed signal contains information about the density of protons across the patient, there is no information about their distribution in the other axis (Fig.17).

Phase-encoding gradients

The phase-encoding gradients are applied for a finite time before the read gradients and perpendicular to them. Their purpose is to apply a phase shift perpendicular to the read gradient to provide spatial information in that direction. Unfortunately, one phase-encoding gradient is insufficient to provide all the data required and a series of phase-encoding gradients are required each one a little stronger than its predecessor. Commonly 64, 128 or 256 are used and if cardiac gating is required the scan time is dictated by the heart rate taking up to 5 minutes (Fig.18).

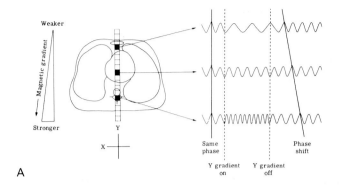

Fig. 18 Phase Encoding. To obtain spatial information in the final direction to enable an image to be constructed, a third gradient (the 'phase encoding' gradient) is applied antero-posteriorly across the patient, i.e. the y direction. **A.** Before the phase encoding gradient is applied, the signals from each column of pixels, because of their position in the x direction, will have the same frequency and the same phase. When the phase encoding gradient is applied, the frequency of the signals at the stronger end of the gradient will be higher than those at the weaker end (Larmor principle). When the gradient is switched off, the frequencies revert back to the same original frequency but have now experienced a 'phase shift'. The degree of phase shift experienced by the signal from each pixel is dependent on both how long the gradient is applied and the position of the pixel in the y

The radio signal produced during each read gradient is a mixture of the effects of the phase signature from the phase-encoding and the read gradients. A low-frequency Fourier transform of the series of different phase shifts due to the phase-encoding gradients gives the spatial information in the plane perpendicular to that from the read gradient.

SEQUENCES

Gating

In the thorax, movement complicates image reconstruction and gating for cardiac and respiratory movement are sometimes needed. Some techniques exist which can overcome part of the image degradation problems caused by movement. These involve either special fast sequences or a re-ordering and re-scaling of images using a respiratory trace to indicate what modifications are necessary to produce a clear image with all the acquisitions registered properly. One technique developed at the Hammersmith Hospital, Respiratory Ordered Phase Encoding (ROPE) can be used to overcome most respiratory artefact.

Gating does not solve all the problems of blurring due to movement. The cardiac cycle is rarely regular. During inspiration, the heart fills more and beats faster than it does during expiration.

---

direction. **B.** To apply the phase encoding gradient once is not enough as this would only provide information for one column of pixels. If no phase encoding gradient is applied, the signals generated in all the pixels in the column will be in phase, as in (**A**) above, and are indicated by all the vector arrows pointing upwards. A number of variable amplitude gradients causes the signal phases to diverge in the y direction by a degree dependent on their position in each gradient. The middle pixel experiences no gradient, pixels above experience a gradient in one direction and pixels below a gradient in the opposite direction. As each gradient is on for a finite time, the phase shifts will be frozen and imprinted on all the signals arriving at the receiver coil below.

After each gradient each pixel in the column will experience the same phase shift. This can readily be seen in the top pixel which after each gradient experiences a 180 degree phase shift as indicated by the vector arrows reading left to right. Note that the middle pixel experiences no phase shift. The output from each pixel over many gradients will modulate the sine and cosine components of the receiver with a different low frequency sine wave, the value of which will depend on the pixels' position relative to the centre of the gradient.

A low frequency Fourier transform of all the amplitudes of the signals over many gradients will assign intensity values to each pixel in the y direction.

The number of phase encoding gradients applied is commonly 128 or 256, with interpolation to derive the intermediate lines if the image is to be displayed on the common 512 matrix. This technique shortens acquisition time.

Respiration is not regular and every few minutes an extra large breath followed by a redistribution of blood and active areas of lung takes place. The effect of both of these irregularities is to degrade images which depend on averaging.

Spin echo and field echo

If the net magnetization in the patient is pushed into the xy axis due to the T1, and the $T2^\star$ effects, the radio signal detected from the patient decreases rapidly. This diminishing signal is known as the free induction decay (FID). The major contributor to the signal loss is the field inhomogeneity $T2^\star$. This loss can be overcome. If the direction in which the net magnetization is spinning is reversed by the application of a radio pulse turning it through an angle of 180 degrees, the forces which were causing the precessions to dephase and the net magnetization to go out of unison are reversed and rephasing will take place producing a signal again. This rephased signal is known as the spin echo (Figs.19–21). This process can be repeated a number of times and

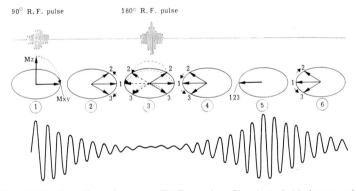

Fig. 19 The Spin Echo Sequence–T2 Dependent Signal. 1. A 90 degree pulse displaces the net magnetization into the xy plane. The protons are all precessing in phase and a large signal is detected. 2. Because of T2 effects some protons will precess faster (**2**) some slower (**3**) and some will remain constant (**1**) with the effect that they precess out of phase and the signal will be lost. 3. If a 180 degree pulse is now delivered, the magnetization will be 'flipped' through 180 degrees. 4. The protons that were precessing faster will now catch up with the slower protons and eventually they will all be precessing at the same rate. 5. As the protons are all in phase once again the detectable signal has now grown in amplitude and forms the 'echo' which is the signal that is used to construct the spin echo images. 6. Once again the protons, due to T2 effects, will fall out of phase and the signal will again be lost.

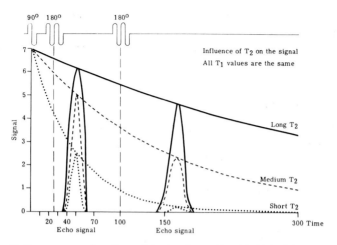

Fig. 20 Demonstrates the effects of altering the position (timing) of the 180 degree pulse in the spin echo sequence to differentiate tissues with different T2 values. If the 180 pulse is delivered at 25 ms, the signal intensity from all three tissues is as shown. However, when the 180 degree pulse is delivered at 100 ms, the signal intensity from the tissue with a short T2 value is very small compared with that from the tissue with a long T2 value which is relatively large.

on each occasion the spin echo is reduced in intensity for three reasons:

(a) The T2* effect causes loss of cohesion
(b) The system is not perfect and the 180 degree radio pulses do not exactly reverse all the spins.

An alternative way of forming an image is to use a radio frequency pulse to invert the nuclei is to leave them precessing in the same direction and to reverse the magnetic field. This is known as a field echo rather than a spin echo. (In the United States, this is usually termed a gradient echo.)

Inversion recovery

An initial 180 degree radio pulse will produce no signal because the net magnetization is in the z direction. After varying times, a 90 degree pulse and spin echo experiments can be carried out. The amplitude of the resultant signal is related to the amount of T1 decay that has taken place during the delay. The echo and repetition times can be varied to emphasise the effects of T1 and T2 and encode tissue characteristics in the MR signal. An example

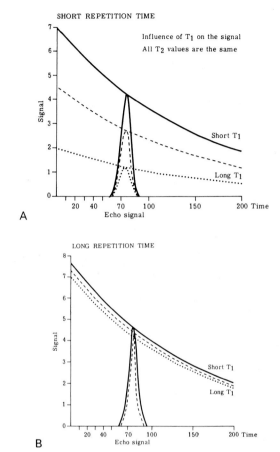

Fig. 21 A. If the time between successive sequences (repetition time) is short, the amount of magnetization that will have relaxed back to equilibrium (Mz) will be different for tissues with differing T1 values. Tissues with a short T1 value will produce a signal of greater intensity when the magnetization is deflected into the xy plane by a 90 degree pulse than the signal produced by tissues with a short T1 value. Tissues with short T1 values can therefore be differentiated from those with long T1 values. **B.** If the repetition time is long, the extent of relaxation back to equilibrium will be near maximum for all tissues, therefore the signal obtained when the magnetization is deflected into the xy plane will be of the same intensity and differentiation between tissues will be lost.

is the separation of fat from sarcoid tissue, both give a bright signal but an inversion recovery sequence using a short interpulse interval—the interpulse interval is denoted by the Greek letter tau (Fig.22).

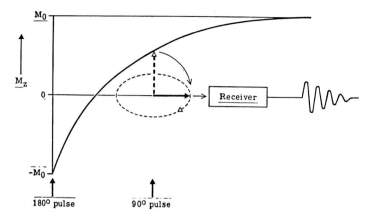

Fig. 22 The Inversion Recovery Sequence–T1 Dependent Signal. Illustrates the signal obtained when a 180 degree pulse is followed by a 90 degree pulse. A 180 degree pulse is first delivered to invert the net magnetization through 180 degrees (from Mz to M − z). At any desired point after the 180 degree pulse, a 90 degree pulse will deflect the magnetization into the xy plane. The intesity of the signal obtained will be dependent on the size of Mz at the time the 90 degree pulse was delivered and therefore on the amount of inversion recovery back to equilibrium due to T1 relaxation.

Sequence to measure blood flow

Several sequences have been developed both to show moving blood as an angio-like picture and to quantify flow. Methods which have been suggested and tried are:

1. Time of flight

The first part of an MR sequence is done in a slice and the remainder of the sequence (obtaining the echo) is done in a second slice downstream in the expected direction of flow. This is difficult to quantify and it has little value, although it can be used in a transverse slice to establish whether a vessel is present or not.

2. The slice saturation technique

If a series of RF pulses are applied frequently to the slice, the direction of the protons will be randomized and there will be no net magnetic vector in any direction. Therefore, a conventional MR sequence can produce no signal. If, after a period of time, a sequence is applied, magnetically clean material flowing into the slice will give a signal. This signal will increase in magnitude as the vessel within the slice is filled. When the segment of vessel is full, the signal which was rising during a series of sequences during the filling phase remains constant. It is possible to obtain an estimate of flow and of the diameter of the vessel. It is difficult to calibrate this technique to give accurate quantitative velocity measurements.

3. Phase mapping

There are three components to the radio signal emanating from a slice which has undergone an MR experiment. These are frequency, amplitude and phase. Velocity can be encoded in the phase of the signal by applying a magnetic gradient for a finite time along the expected direction of flow. The gradient is switched off for a similar period of time and then applied in the opposite direction with a duration exactly corresponding to the original gradient. Material in the body which is not moving will experience two equal and opposite phase changes due to the gradients and there will be zero net phase change. Material which is moving will change its phase territory and will experience a phase change directly proportional to the velocity of flow at each point across a vessel. Unfortunately, there is no technique whereby it is possible to distinguish between a phase change of say, three-quarters of a cycle and one and three-quarters of a cycle or 'n' and three-quarters of a cycle.

4. Field even echo rephasing (FEER)

This sequence was developed at the National Heart and Chest Hospitals by Firmin and Nayler. The shortcomings of simple phase mapping are overcome by allowing moving material to go more than one cycle out of phase at the first echo and applying gradients which will nearly rephase them at the second echo. The advantage of this technique is that there is good signal from the moving fluid, be it arterial blood, venous blood, lymph or fluid in the pleural cavity, pericardium, abscesses, etc., and this signal can be analysed for its phase shift to produce accurate measurements. Subtle changes in the gradients can be used either to produce strong signal and angio-like images or to encode velocity or acceleration.

Detection of atheroma

The generalized presence of atheroma can be established or excluded by measuring aortic compliance or pulse wave velocity in the younger adult. The pulse wave velocity rises with age and compliance falls with age, thus in the older age groups over the age of 50 this is not a reliable screening test. In these patients and in subjects in whom atheroma is suspected, atheromatous plaques can be detected using high resolution transverse or longitudinal sections of the vessels in which the lesions are suspected. When a plaque is found, its significance in the circulation can be established by measuring velocity or acceleration or both past it. Blood accelerates upstream of an obstruction, passes the obstruction at high velocity and decelerates downstream of it. Colour-coded images highlight the lesions which can then be studied in detail.

It is important to know whether an atheromatous plaque is at an early stage when it is mainly smooth muscle and platelets and hopefully reversible, whether it is infiltrated with lipids or whether it is scarred and irreversible. This classification can be done using magnetic resonance techniques which highlight fat or water utilizing the difference in precessional rate between protons in fat and water. The read gradient can be centred so that it will detect one or the other. Subtraction of the fat and water images shows the amount of tissue which contains a mixture of both.

Other sequences

Sequences are being developed to highlight many pathological conditions and it is likely that in the future magnetic resonance machines will be capable of sequences to show most common pathological conditions without the aid of image enhancement.

ACKNOWLEDGEMENTS

The author wishes to thank the Board of Governors of the National Heart and Chest Hospitals and the Coronary Artery Disease Research Association (CORDA) for the backing and financial support for the unique MR unit, which does almost exclusively cardiopulmonary studies, in which the work on which this chapter is based was done.

The work could not have been possible without the scientific and clinical support from Sir Godfrey Hounsfield, Dr. D Firmin, Dr. Simon Rees, Dr. Richard Underwood, Dr. Richard Klipstein, Dr. Raad Mohiaddin, Miss Elisabeth Bruman and Mr. Karl Lotey, all of the MR Unit. Professor Hugo Bogren and Dr. Douglas Lowell on sabbatical years and many others.

Mr. John McNeill understood the problems of explaining MR without resorting to mathematical formulae and with the help of the artistic skills of Miss Lindsey Pegus turned the author's sketches into the series of illustrations in this chapter.

British Medical Bulletin (1989) Vol. 45, No. 4, pp. 881–895
© The British Council 1989

Radionuclide assessment of ventricular function in patients with coronary artery disease: Clinical perspective

D S Dymond
Department of Cardiology, St Bartholomew's Hospital, London, UK

This paper describes how the clinical applications of radionuclide ventriculography have developed during the last decade. The role of resting radionuclide angiography in the assessment of myocardial infarctions, suspected left ventricular aneurysms, and the assessment of right ventricular function are discussed. Currently exercise radionuclide angiography probably represents the best way of assessing left ventricular function under stress. Extensive experience has been gained with this technique in a large number of centres worldwide. Initially the techniques were compared against coronary arteriography as the gold standard, figures for sensitivity, specificity and predictive value of the test in predicting stenosed coronary arteries were produced. This article points out that the exercise study demonstrates the physiological response of the left ventricle to exercise and not every patient with coronary artery disease can be expected to manifest abnormal physiology. Certain valuable prognostic information may be obtained from the results of the exercise radionuclide studies which may guide cardiologists as to which patients should be treated conservatively and which patients should undergo a prognostic intervention. The techniques are of major value in determining the results of both medical and

0007–1420/89/0045–0881/$10.00

interventional therapy. Abnormal ventricular function response to exercise is not specific for coronary artery disease however, and the relevance of the study must be analysed in relationship to the population under investigation.

Radionuclide techniques have been applied to the study of ventricular function across the whole spectrum of coronary artery disease (CAD). At various times during the evolution of nuclear cardiology, their use has been advocated as mass screening techniques in large asymptomatic populations on the one hand, and in the routine assessment of post myocardial infarction patients or post bypass surgery at the other extreme. There is little doubt that the interpretation of the results of these tests in patients with coronary disease has changed during the last decade and they should be regarded as complementary rather than exclusive.[1] Left and right ventricular function may be assessed by either first pass or equilibrium imaging but the non-imaging nuclear probe can only be used to measure left ventricular ejection fraction and relative volumes. The bulk of this paper will refer to the imaging techniques which are more often used in clinical practice.

RESTING STUDIES

Resting radionuclide ventriculograms are often used to measure left ventricular ejection fraction in patients who have suffered acute myocardial infarction or in patients with known coronary artery disease who present with cardiomegaly, symptoms of heart failure, or ventricular arrhythmias. Although some have advocated the routine use of this technique in patients with acute myocardial infarction, a resting study on its own often contributes little to the management of these patients.[2] In patients in whom a large amount of myocardial damage is suspected, however, a radionuclide ejection fraction may help in deciding whether a patient is a candidate for prognostic testing by coronary arteriography. The intimate relationship between left ventricular ejection fraction and prognosis[3] is the rationale for this. Thus a patient who is shown to have an ejection fraction of approximately 20% post-infarction may well be better served by careful monitoring for life-threatening arrhythmias and attention to electrolyte balance, than by coronary arteriography, as revascularization may not enhance prognosis when the left ventricle is severely damaged in this way. Left ventricular aneurysms can be differentiated in many cases from diffusely hypokinetic ventricles[4] which again may influence the decision as to whether to proceeed to invasive investigations. In some patients false aneurysms will be demonstrated which are connected to the left ventricular cavity through a narrow neck and given the tendency of these false aneurysms to rupture, urgent angiography and surgical repair is indicated. The sophistication of modern echo technology has perhaps diminished the role of radionuclide angiography in these situations however as both true and false left ventricular aneurysms can often be detected by ultrasonic means. In addition intracardiac thrombus is not detectable by radionuclide angiography. When the measurement of left ventricular ejection fraction is required the radionuclide technique is probably more accurate.

In recent years much interest has focused upon the right ventricle and its involvement in the ischaemic process. Right ventricular ejection fraction may be depressed either as a consequence of left ventricular dysfunction resulting in pulmonary hypertension, or the ischaemic insult may concentrate more on the right ventricle than the left. This is particularly likely to occur in inferior myocardial infarction.[5] Depression of right ventricular ejection fraction is common in inferior myocardial infarction and right ventricular dysfunction has been recognized to produce a clinical syndrome of a low cardiac output state and hypotension which requires different therapeutic manoeuvres from the syndrome associated with left ventricular dysfunction. Right ventricular dysfunction often recovers however with time in this context.[6]

EXERCISE STUDIES

It is the ability to study ventricular function under stress that has made exercise radionuclide angiography a highly attractive technique in patients with coronary artery disease and has in many respects helped cardiologists to re-think attitudes towards previously accepted gold standards.

It is well known that cardiac function will deteriorate when the organ becomes ischaemic. It is possible to have entirely normal left ventricular function at rest even in the presence of very severe coronary artery disease, but abnormalities of function appear when oxygen demand exceeds supply and this may occur temporally long before the perception of pain, if indeed the latter occurs at all. Historically the first study to demonstrate that abnormalities of global and regional left ventricular function could be detected during exercise in patients with coronary disease was published by Borer et al.[7] This study also described a diametrically opposite response of an increase in ejection fraction in normal individuals. Over the years, however, it has become apparent that not only do normality and abnormality require precise and careful definition, but not all patients who have normal coronary arteries will show a typically normal response to exercise and conversely not all patients with angiographically demonstrated coronary disease will show an abnormal response.

NUCLEAR ANGIOGRAPHY IN THE 'DETECTION' OF CORONARY DISEASE

It was quite common to see such a heading in abstracts and papers during the late 70s and early 1980s. It should be apparent however that only a coronary arteriogram can demonstrate stenoses and occlusions in the coronary tree and that exercise nuclear angiography produces evidence of disturbed global and regional function during exercise, which may or may not reflect ischaemia in the territory supplied by diseased arteries. As long as the coronary arteriogram remained the cardiologist's gold standard for normality or abnormality, then all other tests had to suffer by comparison. Several papers described acceptable sensitivities, specificities and predictive values for the presence or absence of coronary disease using the coronary arteriogram as the reference point.[8-10] A scan which showed a normal ejection fraction response and no inducible regional dysfunction, in a patient with angiographically demonstrated disease, was therefore regarded as 'a false negative'. As will be discussed below, this is perhaps not the correct way of interpreting the results and important information on patients' long term prognosis may well be available from such data. Figure 1 shows the ejection fraction response from rest to exercise along with the double products in a group of 49 male patients with coronary artery disease. Although the mean ejection fraction falls in this group it is evident that several of the patients do not show such a fall. The ejection fraction response and double product response in a group of 15 normal males with a mean age of 33 years is shown in Figure 2, not every patient shows an increase in ejection fraction. In these groups of patients, the criterion of a fall

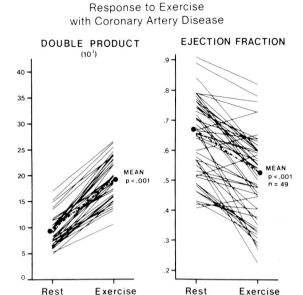

Fig. 1 Rest and exercise double products and rest and exercise ejection fraction response in 49 male patients with documented coronary artery disease.

in ejection fraction produced a 90% sensitivity for coronary disease, but a 73% specificity and a predictive value of 92%. If the criteria for an abnormal ejection fraction response are made more stringent, the specificity may be improved but the sensitivity will be reduced. In this group of patients if a fall in ejection fraction of 8% or more was used to define an abnormal response the sensitivity drops to 63%, but the specificity is 100%. The addition of wall motion abnormality to ejection fraction response will improve sensitivity and in most cases will not lead to a lower specificity. Given that these data come from a selected group of patients undergoing coronary angiography, it is not surprising to learn that in an unselected group of patients presenting with chest pain of uncertain nature the sensitivities and specificities will be lower.[11]

NUCLEAR ANGIOGRAPHY IN THE EXCLUSION OF CORONARY DISEASE

As with thallium perfusion imaging, exercise radionuclide angiography has often been used as an attempt to decide whether to carry

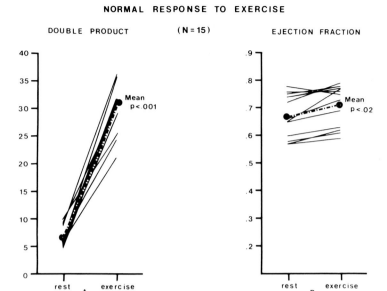

Fig. 2 Rest and exercise double products and rest and exercise ejection fractions in 15 normal healthy males.

out a coronary arteriogram on a patient with angina or atypical chest pain. For reasons outlined above, a normal nuclear angiogram on exercise does not exclude the presence of coronary artery disease, but means that ischaemia cannot be detected on that particular occasion. The relevance of a positive or negative investigation will depend on the prevalence of the disease in the population under study. This concept has been referred to as Bayes' theorem, and is explained in an elegant review by Epstein.[12] In a patient who presents with typical angina pectoris, a negative exercise ECG or a negative exercise radionuclide angiogram do not significantly lessen the likelihood of coronary artery disease being present. Conversely an abnormal nuclear angiogram in a young non-smoking female with sharp stabbing chest pain, does not increase the likelihood of her having coronary artery disease compared to the likelihood before the test was performed, because the prevalence of disease in a similar population would be so low. The exercise nuclear angiogram will contribute most as a pre-catheterisation guide in middle aged patients with atypical chest pain, probably with at least one or more risk factors for coronary disease, in whom the diagnosis of angina is not absolutely confident.[12] An abnormal study will lead to the patient being studied by coronary angiography. Unfortunately this approach is not fool proof. Considerable experience has been gained in the last decade of patients with pain which may be typically or atypically ischaemic in nature, who have abnormal exercise ECGs, abnormal exercise radionuclide angiograms, and yet who have subsequently been found to have normal coronary arteries.[13,14] Some of these patients will subsequently be labelled as 'angina with normal coronary arteries', sometimes known as *Syndrome X*. The fact that so many of these patients will have abnormal radionuclide studies has intensified the investigation of this difficult and challenging group of patients and the aetiology of their pain and of their abnormal studies remains unclear. The condition may well be over-diagnosed, however, and other conditions can produce abnormal responses to exercise in patients who do not have coronary artery disease. These are listed in Table 1.

It is thus evident that an abnormal response in the presence of conditions mentioned in Table 1 must be interpreted in the clinical context. What can be said with some certainty is that a totally normal exercise response in a patient with no evidence of mitral prolapse, hypertension, left bundle branch block etc, may lead to the avoidance of a cardiac catheterisation particularly on prognostic grounds.

DEFINITION OF A NORMAL OR ABNORMAL RESPONSE

The definition of normality and abnormality has produced some lively debate and remains somewhat controversial. Several studies have compared patients with documented coronary disease (the abnormal group) to a variety of 'controls'. The response of the control group dictates what various laboratories regard as normal.

Table 1   Some common conditions which produce abnormal responses to exercise in patients without coronary artery disease

'Syndrome X'
Left bundle branch block
Mitral valve prolapse
Aortic and mitral valve disease
Hypertension
Myopathic disease

However, patients with chest pain who undergo coronary arteriography and have normal coronary arteries may not, as is discussed above, be truly normal. Olympic athletes may be normal but these super-fit individuals hardly represent the average normal individual passing though a busy laboratory. Several factors dictate the normal response to exercise, including the population labelled as normal,[15] the position of exercise (supine or upright),[16] the technology (first pass or equilibrium), the adequacy of exercise[17] the exercise protocol used,[18] the age of the patient,[19] or resting ejection fraction[20] and whether the patient is on medication.[21] There is almost universal agreement therefore that it is the responsibility of each nuclear laboratory to define their own normal responses pertinent to their own populations.

Most normal individuals will increase their ejection fraction during dynamic exercise. This is not universally the case, however, and in the author's experience many normals when imaged at peak exercise using the first pass technique in the upright position will only maintain their ejection fraction at resting levels. Laboratories that image immediately post exercise will nearly always demonstrate a larger rise in ejection fraction than if the study had been carried out at peak exercise.[22] Given the different cameras and computer programmes and the divergent use of first pass or equilibrium imaging, it is not surprising that unanimous agreement on the normal response cannot be achieved.

Volume measurements have been made from radionuclide angiograms[4,23] and changes in volumetric measurement have been used to define normality or abnormality. These have not gained very wide acceptance however for the very good reason that accurate volume determination requires a reliable way of defining the edge of the chamber under investigation, usually the left ventricle. Edge detection is not one of the major strengths of dynamic nuclear imaging and both geometric techniques and non-geometric techniques are flawed.

Regional cardiac function can be assessed either from inspection of a cine loop or from a variety of computer generated images including superimposed contours, regional ejection fraction images, phase images or amplitude images. No one functional image has been proved beyond doubt to be superior to the others and each laboratory will have its own standard for defining normal and abnormal regional function. This has been partly discussed in the chapter on 'Technical introduction to nuclear imaging' (this issue).

QUANTIFICATION OF CORONARY ARTERY DISEASE

Given the intimate relationship between extent of underlying coronary artery disease and prognosis,[24] documented by several studies, it would be useful if radionuclide angiography could indicate whether the patient had single, double or triple vessel disease or even a left main stem stenosis. Several studies have attempted both with thallium scintigraphy and exercise function studies to predict the extent of disease either by the degree of fall in ejection fraction or by the extent of induced wall motion abnormalities. These attempts have not been fruitful however, because of course classification of disease according to the number of arteries involved does not provide any information on the amount of myocardium dependent upon each diseased artery. Attempts to take into account the dominance of a stenosed artery and whether the disease is proximal or distal have produced coronary scores but these too have not been fruitful in classifying individual patients according to their radionuclide response, although groups of patients may show statistically significant differences.[25] Further attempts to take into account the duration of exercise and to relate the fall in ejection fraction to the time taken for the ejection fraction to fall have also produced significant intergroup differences but currently it is not possible to classify an individual accurately in this way.[26] The modern concept is to take into account 'the total ischaemic burden' and it has been realized that a single proximal left anterior descending stenosis may produce the same degree of functional instability or exercise induced ischaemia, as stenoses in three vessels each of which on its own is not so important. The comparison between coronary arteriography and exercise radionuclide angiography has therefore been turned around somewhat and many laboratories would now combine information obtained from the coronary arteriogram and from radionuclide studies to decide whether to intervene on a particular lesion, rather than rely on the coronary arteriogram alone. Plate 2 shows an example of rest and exercise studies from a patient with a single left anterior descending stenosis before and after coronary angioplasty. In this patient the left anterior descending was an extremely important vessel which wrapped around the apex of the left ventricle and supplied part of the inferior wall. The drop in ejection fraction to 26% from 64% indicates a large amount of muscle at risk and, as will be discussed below, this can provide important prognostic information and it may be immaterial whether this abnormality is produced by one single vessel stenosis or triple vessel disease.

ASSESSMENT OF RIGHT VENTRICULAR FUNCTION ON EXERCISE IN CAD

Although by far of the majority of papers have dealt with the left ventricular response to exercise, the principles which apply to assessment of left ventricular function may also be applied to the right ventricle and its ejection fraction may be measured at rest and exercise. Some work had suggested that right ventricular dysfunction on exercise could be used to predict whether the right coronary artery was involved in the atheromatous process[27] and also claims were made about the ability to detect proximal versus distal right coronary stenoses. This has not been confirmed subsequently[28] however and right ventricular function on exercise adds very little to the assessment of patients with coronary artery disease.

ASSESSMENT OF THE RESULTS OF THERAPY

Medical treatment

Several studies have shown that patients with coronary disease who exhibit signs of ischaemia under stress will have improvement or normalization of this response, when the exercise radionuclide study is repeated on various anti-ischaemic agents.[29] The mechanisms by which various drugs achieve such improvement obviously differ from drug to drug.[29] The relevance of these responses will be further discussed below.

Serial testing at 6 monthly or yearly intervals is a valuable aid in monitoring non-invasively the possible progression of coronary disease in patients being treated medically. If the extent of inducible ischaemia, either in terms of the fall in ejection fraction with exercise or the extent of regional asynergy with exercise, increases, this may suggest the patient is entering a high risk prognostic group. Although prospective studies to assess this potential role of radionuclide angiography have not yet been done, the prognostic information from an abnormal radionuclide angiogram which will be discussed below, might make this a logical way in deciding whether to intervene prognostically.

Patients who have undergone either coronary angioplasty or

coronary bypass surgery can be assessed pre and post intervention.[30,31] We have found this technique particularly valuable in
patients who return after coronary angioplasty or bypass surgery
with chest pains of uncertain nature and it would not be our policy
to re-investigate a patient with a normal response to exercise in
this context, unless the history of recurrent angina was clinically
very convincing. Plate 2 shows examples following a successful
angioplasty to the left anterior descending. The techniques also
provide a more objective assessment of the results of the intervention than inspection of the coronary arteriogram and a normal
functional response to exercise following the procedure indicates
adequate revascularization even if the dilated artery looks less than
perfect. The converse is also true in that what may be regarded as a
satisfactory angiographic appearance may in fact not be associated
with normalization of exercise function.

Figure 3 shows ejection fraction response to exercise in the
patients in Figure 2 after coronary bypass surgery. It is apparent
that the mean ejection fraction on exercise as a group has improved,
although some patients still show an abnormal response.

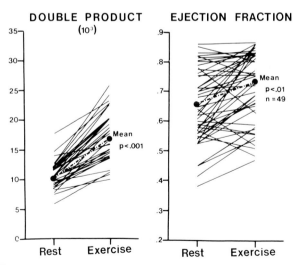

Fig. 3 Rest and exercise double products and ejection fractions in 49 patients after
revascularization surgery. In each graph the means are represented by the large
black circle.

ASSESSMENT OF PROGNOSIS IN CAD

Perhaps the most exciting area currently under investigation is the role of radionuclide angiography in assessing prognosis. Until fairly recently, patients with little or no symptoms would be recommended for revascularization if they had triple vessel disease, some combinations of double vessel disease, or a left main stem stenosis. This has been based on survival studies related to coronary anatomy.[24] Given that the coronary arteriogram is not a physiological measurement, workers have begun to test the hypothesis that the degree of ischaemia induced by exercise might be a more powerful predictor of prognosis in patients with little or no symptoms, than the coronary arteriogram. Jones et al. 1983[32] have shown (a) that survival is not improved by surgery in patients with normal exercise radionuclide angiograms pre-operatively, (b) patients with abnormal responses to exercise fare worse prognostically than patients with normal responses when treated medically, and (c) patients with abnormal radionuclide angiograms have improved survival with surgery than with medical treatment. Although this study suffered some drawbacks, subsequent work has confirmed the finding that certain patients with triple vessel coronary artery disease with normal responses to exercise are in a benign prognostic group over a 5 year follow-up period.[33] The corollary to this is that patients with single vessel disease who demonstrate large amounts of functional ischaemia on exercise cannot necessarily be regarded as having a benign prognosis, therefore should not necessarily be recommended for conservative treatment. This is particularly true of stenoses of the proximal left anterior descending. There are several gaps in the knowledge, however, that need to be filled before this can be applied with certainty on a prospective basis in the clinical arena. For example, it needs to be demonstrated clearly that patients with single vessel disease who show an abnormal response to exercise should have prognostic interventions, and the relevance of abnormal response off therapy which subsequently normalize on medical therapy is not yet known. In addition some of the events which produce infarction or death, such a plaque rupture, may in fact be unpredictable. Nevertheless it is of interest to those who have worked for sometime in this field to note that the radionuclide studies are now being used to judge the coronary arteriogram which is a reversal of what has happened over the last 10 years.

THE NON-IMAGING NUCLEAR PROBE

This technique which has been mentioned under the Technology Section, is not really designed for widespread clinical use because of the lack of regional information. Ejection fraction and relative volumes can be measured on exercise from the beat-by-beat curves and the effect of anti-ischaemic medication can also be assessed.[34] This does remain currently a research tool however.

Non-dynamic exercise

Alternatives to dynamic exercise have been suggested for laboratories that do not have a suitable exercise facility, or in patients who are physically unable to exercise. The two techniques that have been assessed are firstly the cold pressor technique in which the forearm is immersed in water at approximately 4 degrees centigrade; this has been used particularly with gated equilibrium studies for the demonstration of reversible ischaemia.[35] The changes may be fairly transitory however[36] and current opinion is that this technique is probably not sensitive or specific enough to replace dynamic exercise. The other method involves isometric hand grip[37] which again appeared promising but is no substitute for dynamic exercise.

CONCLUSION

The role of exercise radionuclide angiography has changed during the last 10 years. It is now inappropriate perhaps to regard it as a substitute for coronary arteriography; as a complementary technique for assessing the left ventricular functional response to exercise in ischaemic heart disease, it is probably superior to other techniques currently available. In some cases the results have confused us, e.g. in *Syndrome X*, but in others the demonstration of an ischaemic response has clarified potentially unclear arteriographic data. The assessment of prognosis is probably the most exciting territory under investigation with this technique.

REFERENCES

1 Gutman J, Rozanski A, Garcia E, Maddahi J, Miyamoto A, Berman D. Complementary roles of scintigraphic and angiographic technique in assessment of the extent of coronary artery disease. Am Heart J 1982; 104: 653–660
2 Handler CE, Ellam SV, Maisey MN, Sowton E. Use of an exercise QRS score and radionuclide left ventricular ejection fraction in assessing prognosis after myocardial infarction. Eur Heart J 1987; 8: 243–253

3 Norris RM, Barnaby PF, Brandt PWT et al. Prognosis after recovery from first acute myocardial infarction: determinants of re-infarction and sudden death. Am J Cardiol 1984; 53: 408–413

4 Dymond DS, Jarrit PH, Britton KE, Spurrell RAJ. Detection of post infarction left ventricular aneurysms by first pass radionuclide ventriculography using a multicrystal gamma camera. Br Heart J 1979; 41: 68–78

5 Caplin JL, Dymond DS, Flatman WD, Spurrell RAJ. Global and regional right ventricular function after acute myocardial infarction: dependents upon site of left ventricular infarction. Br Heart J 1987; 58: 101–109

6 Steel P, Kirch D, Ellis J, Vogel R, Battock D. Prompt return to normal of depressed right ventricular ejection fraction in acute inferior infarction. Br Heart J 1977; 39: 1319–1323

7 Borer JS, Bacharach SL, Greene MV, Kent KM, Epstein SE, Johnston GS. Real-time radionuclide cine angiography in the non-invasive evaluation of global and regional left ventricular function at rest and during exercise in patients with coronary artery disease. N Engl J Medicine 1977; 296: 839–844

8 Jengo JA, Freeman R, Brizendine M, Mena I. Detection of coronary artery disease: comparison of exercise stress radionuclide angiocardiography and thallium stress perfusion scanning. Am J Cardiol 1980; 45: 535–541

9 Newman GF, Rerych SK, Upton MT, Sabiston DC, Jones RH. Comparison of electrocardiographic and left ventricular functional changes during exercise. Circulation 1980; 60: 1204–1211

10 Gibbons RJ, Morris KG, Lee K, Colman RE, Cobb FR. Assessment of regional left ventricular function using gated radionuclide angiography. Am J Cardiol 1984; 54: 294–300

11 Austin EH, Cobb FR, Colman RE, Jones RH. Prospective evaluation of radionuclide angiocardiography for the diagnosis of coronary artery disease. Am J Cardiol 1982; 50: 1212–1216

12 Epstein SE. Implications of probability analysis on the strategy used for non-invasive detection of coronary artery disease. Am J Cardiol 1980; 46: 491–499

13 Berger HJ, Sands MJ, Davies RA et al. Exercise left ventricular performance in patients with chest pain, ischaemic-appearing exercise electrocardiograms, and angiographically normal coronary arteries. Ann Intern Med 1981; 94: 186–191

14 Gibbons RJ, Lee KL, Cobb F, Jones RH. Ejection fraction response to exercise in patients with chest pain and normal coronary arteriograms. Circulation 1981; 64: 952–957

15 Bar-Shlomo BZ, Druck MN, Morch JE et al. Left ventricular function in trained and untrained healthy subjects. Circulation 1982; 65: 484–488

16 Poliner LR, Dehmer GJ, Lewis SE, Parkey RW, Blomqvist CG, Willerson JT. Left ventricular performance in normal subjects: a comparison of the responses to exercise in the upright and supine positions. Circulation 1980; 62: 528–534

17 Brady TG, Thrall JH, Lo K, Pitt B. The importance of adequate exercise in the detection of coronary heart disease by radionuclide ventriculography. J Nucl Med 1980; 21: 1125–1130

18 Foster C, Dymond DS, Anholm JD, Pollock ML, Schmidt DH. Effect of exercise protocol on the left ventricular response to exercise. Am J Cardiol 1983; 51: 859–864

19 Port S, Cobb FR, Colman RE, Jones RH. Effect of age on the response of the left ventricular ejection fraction to exercise. N Engl J Med 1980; 303: 1133–1137

20 Port S, McEwan P, Cobb FR, Jones RH. Influence of resting left ventricular function on the left ventricular response to exercise in patients with coronary artery disease. Circulation 1981; 63: 856–863

21 Marshall RC, Wisenberg G, Schelbert HR, Henze E. Effect of oral propranolol on rest, exercise and post exercise left ventricular performance in normal

subjects and in patients with coronary artery disease. Circulation 1981; 63: 572–583

22 Dymond DS, Foster C, Grenier RP, Carpenter J, Schmidt DH. Peak exercise and immediate post exercise imaging for the detection of left ventricular functional abnormalities in coronary artery disease. Am J Cardiol 1984; 53: 1532–1537

23 Kronenberg MW, Parrish MD, Jenkins DW et al. Accuracy of radionuclide ventriculography for estimation of left ventricular volume changes and end-systolic pressure-volume relations. J Am Coll Cardiol 1985; 6: 1064–1072

24 De Rouen TA, Hammermeister KE, Dodge HT. Comparisons of the effects on survival after coronary artery surgery in sub groups of patients from the Seattle Heart Watch. Circulation 1981; 63: 537–545

25 Stone DL, Dymond DS, Elliott AT, Britton KE, Banim SO, Spurrell RAJ. Exercise first pass radionuclide ventriculography in detection of patients with coronary artery disease. Br Heart J 1980; 44: 208–214

26 Caplin JL, Dymond DS, O'Keefe JC et al. Relation between coronary anatomy and serial changes in left ventricular function on exercise: a study using first pass radionuclide angiography with gold-195m. Br Heart J 1986; 55: 120–128

27 Johnson LL, McCarthy DM, Sciacca RR, Cannon PJ. Right ventricular ejection fraction during exercise in patients with coronary artery disease. Circulation 1979; 60: 1284–1291

28 Berger HJ, Johnstone DE, Sands JM, Gottschalk A, Zaret BL. Response of right ventricular ejection fraction to upright bicycle exercise in coronary disease. Circulation 1979; 60: 1292–1300

29 Nestico PF, Hakki A-H, Iskandrian AS. Effects of cardiac medications on ventricular performance: emphasis on evaluation with radionuclide angiography. Am Heart J 1985; 109: 1070–1084

30 Hellman CK, Kamath ML, Schmidt DH, Anholm J, Blau F, Johnson WD. Improvement in left ventricular function after myocardial revascularisation: assessment by first pass rest and exercise nuclear angiography. J Thorac Cardiovasc Surg 1980; 79: 645–655

31 DePuey EG, Leatherman LL, Leachman RD et al. Restenosis after transluminal coronary angioplasty detected with exercise-gated radionuclide ventriculography. J Am Coll Cardiol 1984; 4: 1103–1113

32 Jones RH, Floyd RD, Austin EH, Sabiston DC. The role of radionuclide angiocardiography in the pre-operative prediction of pain relief and prolonged survival following coronary artery bypass grafting. Ann Surg 1983; 197: 743–753

33 Bonow RO, Kent KM, Rosing DR et al. Exercise-induced ischaemia in mildly symptomatic patients with coronary artery disease and preserved left ventricular function: identification of sub-groups at risk of death during medical therapy. N Engl J Med 1984; 311: 1339–1345

34 Caruana M, Jones R, Lahiri A et al. A comprehensive clinical validation of the nuclear stethoscope. Nucl Med Commun 1986; 7: 717–728

35 Wainwright RJ, Brennand-Roper DA, Cueni TA, Sowton E, Hilson AJW, Maisey MN. Cold pressor test in detection of coronary heart disease and cardiomyopathy using technetium-99m gated blood pool imaging. Lancet 1979; ii: 320–323

36 Dymond DS, Caplin JL, Flatman W, Burnett P, Banim S, Spurrell R. Temporal evolution of changes in left ventricular function induced by cold pressor stimulation: an assessment with radionuclide angiography and gold 195m. Br Heart J 1984; 51: 557–564

37 Bodenheimer MM, Banka VS, Fooshee CM, Gillespie JA, Helfant RH. Detection of coronary heart disease using radionuclide determined regional ejection fraction at rest and during hand grip exercise: correlation with coronary arteriography. Circulation 1978; 58: 640–648

British Medical Bulletin (1989) Vol. 45, No. 4, pp. 896–921

Perfusion imaging

A C Tweddel
W Martin
I Hutton
University Department of Medical Cardiology, Royal Infirmary, Glasgow, UK

The term perfusion has varied connotations in different situations.

The word perfusion comes from the Latin to pour or diffuse through or over. Myocardial perfusion depends on (a) coronary artery or vessel flow, and (b) myocardial or muscle flow. The factors which determine perfusion at rest and during stress in coronary vessels and within the myocardium are clearly related but not with a predictable linear relationship.

In animals there is extensive literature concerning the regulation of coronary flow and perfusion obtained by many sophisticated methods. In contrast, the techniques that are applicable to humans are relatively crude. To date, the clinical data available suggests that the normal control of coronary flow in man and in dogs is fairly similar but that models of pathology in animals bear little relation to the compensatory changes found in the coronary circulation in man.[1-3] Although the data available is limited and subject to many technical inaccuracies, this article is confined to the assessment of myocardial perfusion in clinical practice.

MEASUREMENT OF CORONARY FLOW

Coronary sinus thermodilution

This is probably the most widely applied technique for the measurement of coronary flow and was introduced by Ganz et al.[4] This technique has major technical limitations,[5] particularly as it measures flow from an unknown mass of myocardium with an individually variable venous drainage. It is however useful in the individual patient where directional change can be determined in response to pharmacological challenge.

0007–1420/89/0045–0896/$10.00

Arteriographic based measurements of coronary flow

Coronary arteriogram

The most widespread method of indirectly imaging coronary flow is undoubtedly the coronary arteriogram. Decisions are made as to patient management, based on the visual assessment of lesions. 'Quantitative' approaches have been reported by several groups in trying to deal with the inter- and intra-observer variations of clinical estimates. Measurements of minimal stenosis diameter, no matter how carefully performed, are still subject to considerable error.[6] These inaccuracies are further compounded if minimal stenosis is expressed as a percentage of 'normal' diameter, that is a segment of coronary artery adjacent to the stenosis that appears to the observer to be normal. This approach is completely unreliable[7,8] as the adjacent artery which may appear to be normal is often involved in the atherosclerotic process,[9] and can be involved in compensatory changes within the artery wall[10] or be subject to vasoactive or morphological arterial changes.[11] Beatt et al[11] used an absolute measurement of minimum stenosis diameter to avoid these problems with a change >0.72 mm being considered significant, based on twice the variability (0.36 mm ± 1 standard deviation of the mean of the difference between duplicate measurements) and an interpolated reference diameter. It is conceptually attractive to avoid the problem of lesion geometry and single diameter measurements by using absolute area measurements at the point of maximum narrowing. This measurement suffers from the uncertainty of what would be the 'normal' area expected at that point, given that anatomically the arterial tree narrows from base to apex and this will vary with a wide variety of factors such as sex, body size, ventricular hypertrophy, etc. Expressing the area measurements in terms of percentage reduction in luminal cross sectional area again involves the use of adjacent 'normal' arterial segments with all the limitations delineated above.

Given the limitations of measuring stenosis severity arteriographically, the functional significance of a lesion can often not be assessed from the arteriogram alone. This has been clearly demonstrated by the experimental work of Gould.[12] There is a complex, non linear relationship between the pressure gradient across a stenosis and flow, so that the effective resistance of a lesion varies widely with small changes in luminal diameter, once this has been reduced by approximately 70%.[13] And indeed it is in this region of moderate to severe (50–90%) diameter narrowing that it is generally agreed that arteriographic measurements have the greatest limitation. For example, for a fixed level of flow the pressure gradient across a concentric stenosis doubles as percentage luminal diameter narrowing increases from 70 to 80% and doubles again as stenosis increases from 80 to 90%. In contrast, if flow increases through a fixed stenosis, this will enhance the pressure drop across the lesion as a consequence of the normal vasodilatory stimulus (providing aortic pressure is virtually unchanged). Therefore, although flow may increase in the epicardial vessel, subendocardial flow may well fall with subsequent ischaemia. The length and shape of a lesion are as important as cross-sectional area in determining the hydraulic consequences of a stenosis.[14,15] As the degree and severity of a stenosis increases, increasing impedance is compensated for by arteriolar 'reserve' vasodilatation. The ability of the coronary circulation to maintain flow with decreasing coronary pressure must reach a point when autoregulatory vasodilatation is maximal and flow 'reserve' becomes exhausted. The measurement of flow reserve is conceptually attractive in that it combines a measurement both of the stenotic lesion and also the effect on the myocardial bed subtended. However the accurate measurement and interpretation of flow reserve in individual patients in varying conditions is as yet of limited clinical value. This particularly applies to the question as to whether the flow reserve which can be recruited pharmacologically equates to that produced by ischaemia. A discussion as to the theoretical difficulties and limitations of vasodilatory reserve are outwith the scope of this article but is well covered by Klocke and Hoffman.[16–18] Undoubtedly, in time, the advantages of noninvasive imaging with positron emitters, or other perfusion markers, to determine the 'functional' impact of stenosis in terms of impaired coronary flow reserve will become of considerable clinical relevance.

Densitometry and digital subtraction angiography

The first clinical applications of video-densitometry by Rutishauser et al[19] and Smith et al.[20] concentrated on the transit time of dye travelling through vein grafts. When applied to coronary vessels, the accuracy of measurements of transit time is seriously limited by the small calibre, complex course with multiple branches. A new approach using ultrafast computed tomography is very promising and is discussed by Lipton in this issue.

A modification of the videodensitometric method, in association with digital subtraction angiography[21] measures the contrast transit time in the myocardium. However it is impossible to measure absolute flow and it is only suitable for assessing changes in perfusion. The accuracy of the technique is influenced by the method and volume of contrast injected, the effects of the contrast itself on flow and the algorithms chosen to compute the changes in perfusion.[22]

Flow probes and Doppler

Electromagnetic flow probes have been used mainly to assess graft flow. If these are placed intra-operatively, calibration presents a major problem. To assess native vessel flow the artery must be dissected free which can be hazardous and has severely limited the use of flow probes.

Doppler, especially pulsed Doppler which can both send and receive a signal, has obvious advantages. Several studies have shown that changes in velocity accurately reflect changes in flow as measured by microspheres[23] and flow probes.[24] The disadvantages of the Doppler technique are that velocity is measured rather than flow and it is assumed that the cross-sectional area of the vessel examined remains fixed. However this technique has produced interesting results in assessing both reactive hyperaemia and coronary flow reserve in normal vessels,[24] the effects of hypertrophy[2] and has demonstrated the major limitations associated with percentage stenosis in the assessment of physiological significance of coronary lesions.[25,26] More recently catheters have been developed with Doppler crystals attached which, when placed in the coronary artery, can record instantaneous velocity in response to vasodilation,[27] the most recently available being a small 3F catheter which is thought not to cause obstruction in the major coronary vessels and may be able to assess individual coronary obstructions.[28]

'Myocardial' flow

In animals, regional flow to separate layers of the myocardium can be assessed for any instant in time, by the injection of microspheres into the left atrium or left ventricle. No comparable technique is available for humans. A wide variety of labelled microspheres have been used such as technetium-99, indium-133, gadolinium-63, gadolinium-62 and carbon-11, labelled to albumin[29-31] but this provides distribution of flow within the myocardium rather than a regional measure of flow, or indeed differentiation between epicardial and endocardial distribution.

Eckenhoff et al.[32] in 1948 described a method of measuring coronary flow based on the principle that an inert gas (nitrous oxide) diffuses across the capillary membrane in proportion to the rate of coronary blood flow, and the the concentration curve can be obtained from sampling from the coronary sinus which allows calculation of myocardial flow by applying the Fick principle. Several different gases have been employed (H-2 helium, argon and radioactive xenon-133) and with each arterial and/or coronary venous sampling is required to construct desaturation curves. Accurate measurements require stable conditions and a knowledge of the time course of interventions, so that measurements obtained by gas clearance can be timed. These measurements become less reliable if the ventricular myocardium is inhomogeneous (such as during ischaemia or with fibrosis) and suffer from all the limitations previously outlined for coronary sinus thermodilution flow.

An interesting technique proposed by Cibulski et al.[33] involves retrograde coronary venous injection of Krypton-85 during partial closure of the coronary sinus to provide 'hot spot imaging' of the ischaemic area, but again this is really only applicable to the left anterior descending coronary artery territory.

The first assessments of global myocardial flow with external praecordial counting were developed by Herd et al.[34] for Krypton-85 and Ross et al.[35] for xenon-133. Following direct intracoronary injection the gas, dissolved in saline, rapidly diffuses into the myocardium subtended by the artery and is washed out in proportion to the blood flow through the tissue. By using tracers that emit gamma radiation this can be detected externally using a gamma camera and the radioisotope washout curves can be analysed by applying a monoexponential model to the initial slope, according to the Kety formula.[36]

$$\frac{F}{W} = \frac{K \lambda 100}{\rho}$$

where F is the myocardial flow rate per 100 g myocardium which equals W

λ the myocardium to blood partition coefficient (obtained by Conn in normal dog 0.72)[37]

ρ the specific gravity of heart (1.05).

The rate constant K is calculated by

$$K = \frac{\ln 2}{t\,1/2}$$

where t 1/2 is the time in minutes required for the count rate to be reduced by 50%.

This method has been applied by various groups in the United States[38-40] and Europe[41,42] to measure regional flow within the myocardium. In addition to providing dynamic information, with the washout curves reflecting myocardial blood flow, the distribution of the flow can be imaged. The scans shown in Plate 3 demonstrate distribution images for two normal situations, both patients having arteriographically normal vessels; one having a right dominant system with a large right coronary artery, and the other being left dominant. These scans have been obtained at separate times following direct injection of xenon-133 dissolved in saline into the left and then the right coronary artery. Images were acquired using a gamma camera, fitted with a high sensitivity biplane collimator, to provide simultaneous 30° and 70° left anterior oblique projections. High speed frames (initially one second, then five second frames) have been summated and the right coronary artery coded red and the left coronary injection coded green.

Data is processed using a computer with washout curves being constructed from peak to 30 seconds for each of eight regions of interest drawn over the left ventricle and three over the right ventricle. With successive measurements, background activity acquired immediately prior to the injection is subtracted. The repeatability of this technique is $\pm 2\%$ (n = 20) and this correlates well with the reproducibility reported by Engel,[43] the regression equation for 118 regions being $r = 0.903$. As 95% of xenon is excreted in the lungs, measurements may be made repeatedly to assess the effects of pharmacological and physical interventions with a low radiation dose to the patient. At present this is the only technique available which provides a measure of regional myocardial flow using a standard gamma camera.

The limitations of the xenon technique have been extensively described[38,43-45] and these include the physical properties of the tracer, theoretical limitations of the analysis technique and technical constraints.

Xenon-133 has several advantages: it is 'chemically inert, physiologically inactive and highly diffusable'[38] and washout has been shown to be a function of tissue capillary blood flow. Among its disadvantages are the low energy gamma emission (81 keV), which although providing easy collimation and low patient radiation dose, also produces significant Compton scatter (approximately 12.5% at 1.5 cm).[46] Alternative tracers that might be considered include 125-iodoantipyrine which is fat insoluble but recirculates extensively, krypton-85 which has a higher energy gamma emission (but also a beta emission), and O–15 labelled water which has a very short half life. One of the major disadvantages of xenon-133 is that it is very fat soluble, the partition coefficient for fat being 8 while that for myocardium is usually taken as 0.72. This means that since the regional composition of myocardium cannot be determined, and may vary regionally, the partition coefficient in the Kety equation may well vary in an indeterminate way.

The major limitations of the analysis technique are dependent on the inhomogeneity of flow within the myocardium and recirculation of the tracer. Alternative analysis techniques, which avoid assumptions as to homogeneity of myocardial flow, such as multiple exponential analysis[39,40,47] and the height over area method of Zierler[48] require quantitative assessment of later portions of the washout curve, which are most affected by tracer accumulation in epicardial fat and recirculation. The initial 30 seconds of the washout curve is least affected by non-myocardial counts and although this and recirculation are still claimed to have a significant effect,[49] certainly at flow rates under 200 ml/100 g/min flow correlates well with experimental flow measured by a probe.[34,35,43] However, where the myocardium is inhomogeneous, such as when fibrous tissue and viable cells are interspersed, flow rates in that area will be weighted in favour of the higher flow through the normal tissue, and of course this technique in common with all other applied in man can not differentiate epicardial and endocardial flow. The geometrical limitations are common to all two dimensional imaging with the spherical shape of the heart resulting in superimposition of normal and underperfused segments within any single region of interest. This problem is partially resolved by the use of biplane collimation.

Despite these limitations, although exact quantification of regional flow may be suspect, where regional differences in flow are demonstrated this technique has added to our understanding of the pathophysiological changes within the myocardium.

NORMAL FLOW

Total left ventricular flow has been quoted as an average of 61 ml/100 g/min by Cannon[37] and 65.9 ml/100 g/min by Engel[41] (n = 39) and in our laboratory for patients with angiographically normal arteries,[50] comparison of the individual coronary artery distributions are shown below in Table 1.

By using the technique of superimposition of distribution images (Plate 3), the areas of overlap (yellow) indicate areas of dual blood supply. By drawing a region of interest around the left ventricular myocardium and expressing the distribution of each major coronary vessel, as a percentage of this area, the overlap appears to be approximately 50%, and appears particularly in the infero-posterior territory.

In nine patients with arteriographically normal right dominant coronary systems and normal left ventricular function, xenon-133 was injected into each major vessel during two levels of atrial pacing (90 beats/minute and 110 beats/minute) and immediately post maximal symptom limited supine exercise. The change in the percentage of the left ventricle supplied varied only by a maximum of $\pm 8\%$, although the changes in flow calculated from the washout curves suggest that during stress most of the increase in left ventricular flow is supplied by the left coronary artery. This is demonstrated in Table 2.

Table 1 Normal myocardial flow (ml/100 g/min)

	LV	LAD	Cx	RCA (LV)
Cannon	$61.0 \pm 8\%$	63.0%	61.0%	–
Engel	65.9 ± 17.8	64.4 ± 13.9	66.3 ± 17.3	69.1 ± 14.3
G.R.I.	75.5 ± 8.8	76.1 ± 9.1	76.1 ± 11.7	67.5 ± 19.1

Table 2 Percentage changes in flow with atrial pacing and dynamic exercise

	AP 90 beats/min	AP 110 beats/min	Immed. Post Ex.
LV	$14.3 \pm 2.0\%$ *	$45.8 \pm 16\%$ *	$18.5 \pm 5\%$ +
LAD	13.0 ± 2.0 *	40.0 ± 1.0 *	18.0 ± 7 *
Cx	16.0 ± 3.6 *	51.0 ± 14.6 *	24.0 ± 6 *
RCA	-3.6 ± 1.0	$+0.4 \pm 2.0$	$-18 \pm 5\%$

*P < 0.02   +P < 0.05

CORONARY ARTERY DISEASE

At rest, flow measured by xenon washout is not compromised unless the coronary vessel has a sub-total or total obstruction (Plate 4). This is in keeping with other published reports[51,52] and with the absence of chest pain and ischaemia at rest. Engel[43] has demonstrated that post-stenotic flow is not significantly reduced in patients with normal wall motion irrespective of the severity of the coronary obstruction. Patients with lesions >75% with normal wall motion had collaterals present and the normal flow rates were thought to reflect the adequacy of the collaterals (Plate 4). In contrast, flow was reduced to akinetic (40–55%) or hypokinetic (15–30%) left ventricular wall areas, and thus it is difficult to separate the effects of vessel stenosis and left ventricular anatomy. Even in patients with electrocardiographic evidence of infarction, the washout from the akinetic area was at least 10 times faster than that recorded from fibrous tissue or fat at the time of surgery.[53] Thus, it would appear that scar is not the only explanation for reduced xenon washout in akinetic areas. The presence of viable myocardium in akinetic areas, shown both macroscopically and microscopically at the time of surgery and postmortem[54,55] and the presence of only mild fibrosis, with the capacity to increase flow following vasodilator therapy, is in keeping with the hypothesis that regional underperfusion represents both the cause and effect of ventricular asynergy.

COLLATERALS

The contrast angiogram can only delineate vessels down to 50–100 microns and many collateral channels are smaller than this. Collateral channels may not be demonstrated at rest, but may be recruited in response to a changing haemodynamic situation, as has been shown by Rentrop et al.[56] following angioplasty and Matsuda[57] in patients with coronary artery spasm. Because of the small molecular size of xenon-133, it can demonstrate distribution to areas of the left ventricle beyond angiographic resolution. In a group of 50 patients at the time of angiography we have demonstrated[58] that the presence of collateral flow which is capable of responding to exercise (Table 3) is associated with preserved regional wall motion, as measured by percentage shortening (Table 4). This applied whether collaterals were identified either angiographically or by xenon distribution alone (Plate 5).

Table 3 Collateral flow on exercise (ml/100g/min)

Identification	Exercise response	Rest	Exercise	n	p
Angiogram	Increase	43.7 ± 3.4	66.6 ± 8.5	13	< 0.005
Xenon	Increase	30.2 ± 7.9	57.5 ± 9.3	11	< 0.005
Angiogram	Maintained	45.7 ± 5.3	44.7 ± 6.3	6	NS
Xenon	Maintained	39.0 ± 7.6	38.4 ± 3.3	9	NS
Angiogram	Decreased	50.3 ± 7.6	35.5 ± 7.4	6	< 0.05
Xenon	Decreased	47.5 ± 6.4	24.7 ± 5.9	10	< 0.01

Table 4 Left ventricular function

Collaterals Identified	Angiographically	Xenon	Both
Collateral flow on exercise		*Ejection Fraction %*	
Increased	37.5 ± 2.6	45.7 ± 2.9	37.9 ± 2.5
Maintained	50.2 ± 2.8	39.1 ± 2.7	42.1 ± 2.5
Decreased	34.0 ± 2.0	41.0 ± 2.0	38.4 ± 2.7
		Percentage Shortening %	
Increased	35.0 ± 8.2★	43.5 ± 6.0★	38.9 ± 3.9★
Maintained	45.7 ± 9.3★★	34.2 ± 6.6★	38.8 ± 4.0★
Increased and Maintained	39.8 ± 8.8★★	38.9 ± 6.3★	38.8 ± 2.8★★
Decreased	18.5 ± 6.1	29.9 ± 3.0	25.6 ± 2.8

★$P < 0.05$
★★$P < 0.001$

PHARMACOLOGICAL INTERVENTION

Glyceryl trinitrin

Engel[43] showed that 0.8 mg of sublingual glyceryl trinitrin caused a decrease in mean arterial pressure from 96 to 86 mmHg and increased the heart rate from 71 to 79 beats/minute. Highly significant decreases in flow were noted in normal and post-stenotic areas (-6.8% and -13.8% respectively) suggesting that the prophylactic effects of nitroglycerin results from decreased myocardial oxygen consumption rather than an increase in flow.

In 35 patients given a metered dose of 0.4 mg of sublingual nitrate, insignificant haemodynamic changes occurred (heart rate 63.5 ± 2 to 65.1 ± 3 beats/minute) and mean arterial pressure 87 ± 3 to 80 ± 3 mmHg). In regions supplied by arteriographically normal vessels, flow tended to increase (LAD + 7%, Cx + 9%,

Table 5 'Collateral flow' ml/100g/min

Distribution	n	Mean flow at rest	Mean flow on exercise
LCA	8	23.1 ± 5.7	40.4 ± 11.3
RCA	10	52.7 ± 6.1	66.6 ± 7.2
Cx	4	35.5 ± 7.0	30.3 ± 13.1
MEAN	22	38.8 ± 6.3	50.5 ± 10.5
With Nitrate			
LCA	7	29.4 ± 3.8	22.4 ± 5.6
RCA	12	40.2 ± 4.8	59.8 ± 6.7 P < 0.05
Cx	3	33.0 ± 8.5	34.3 ± 5.0
MEAN	22	35.8 ± 5.7	43.3 ± 5.9

Response to Exercise

Distribution	n	Control	n	With Nitrate
Mean difference in flow (ml/100g/min) increasing on exercise				
LAD	6	29.3 ± 12.6	3	9.3 ± 2.8
RCA	7	24.7 ± 6.3	9	28.4 ± 4.2
Cx	1	32	1	15
MEAN		27.2 ± 11.6		23.0 ± 4.8
Mean difference in flow (ml/100g/min) falling with exercise				
LAD	2	19.0 ± 9.0	4	19.3 ± 4.7
RCA	3	11.3 ± 5.0	3	7.0 ± 3.0
Cx	3	17.7 ± 9.0	2	6.5 ± 2.5
MEAN		15.6 ± 7.8		12.4 ± 3.4

RCA + 23%) but in regions supplied by arteries with high grade occlusion flow fell significantly (LAD − 19% $P < 0.01$; RCA − 17% $P < 0.01$; Cx − 7%) and regions supplied by collaterals fell more significantly (-27% $P < 0.05$). Similar results were found when glyceryl trinitrate was given immediately post exercise for the relief of angina and regional flow data compared to that of after a control exercise test in 16 male patients. In general, areas of normal flow increased whereas in jeopardized area flow tended to decrease (Table 5). However occasionally the areas of distribution changed (Plate 6).

Beta blockers

Similar results were found by Engel[43] following atenolol administration, with flow decreasing both to normal (-13%) and abnormal or post-stenotic areas (-17%) both in regions with and without left ventricular asynergy, confirming that for atenolol a decrease in myocardial oxygen consumption rather than an increase in coronary flow is the mechanism of action.

Vasodilators

The calcium channel blocker nifedipine appears to have a different action. 20 mg given by Engel produced a small decrease in mean arterial pressure (95–87 mmHg) and a 20% fall in coronary vascular resistance, with a heart rate increase from 79 to 80 beats/minute. Flow increased in normal ($+11\%$ $P<0.05$) and post-stenotic areas ($+18\%$ $P<0.05$). Using 10 mg of sublingual nifedipine we have found similar increases in flow and in particular the collateral flow which increases (mean $+20\%$ $P<0.01$). Given intracoronary nifedipine may increase flow by as much as 200% which is similar to the effects seen with intracoronary papaverine.

MECHANICAL INTERVENTION

Bypass grafts

One of the areas where xenon may provide unique information is the assessment of graft function. With direct intra-graft injection, the subsequent scans provide a measure of the distribution to the myocardium in addition to the flow through the myocardium from the washout curves. Arteriographic patency does not guarantee either normal distribution of the graft (this depends on the disease in the vessel grafted) or indeed normal myocardial washout. Plate 7 demonstrates a large patent right coronary artery graft with poor clearance from the left ventricular myocardium.

In a small group of internal mammary grafts placed to the left anterior descending we found that in 10 patients flow increased in the myocardium in response to the stress of atrial pacing (46.2 ± 5.4 to 55.1 ± 5.3 ml/100 g/min, atrial pacing 120 beats/minute) while in 10 flow decreased (45.6 ± 4.7 to 38.4 ± 6 ml/100 g/min, atrial pacing 120 beats/minute, $P<0.05$). The only difference between the groups that could be identified was that where flow increased, the internal mammary graft was of a similar size or smaller than the native left anterior descending coronary artery whereas where flow fell the graft was larger than the native vessel.

Positron emission tomography

With the recent improvement in technology of PET imaging and the resolution in the order of 4 mm, improved image quality and faster dynamic imaging with cardiac gating, the advantages of PET imaging appear to be that it can detect far more subtle changes in flow than any other technique. This is particularly true when the information is combined from a flow marker such as [^{13}N]-ammonia or ^{82}Rb with metabolic markers such as FDG [^{18}F]-fluorodeoxy-D-glucose). PET[30] perfusion imaging would be more logically considered with imaging of myocardial metabolism which will be discussed later in this volume.

Flow and myocardial uptake

Thallium-201 is the most widely used imaging agent for perfusion and is useful not only in detecting the presence of coronary artery disease but also for the assessment of interventions, myocardial viability, infarct sizing and assessment of prognosis.

Technical considerations

The development and more widespread application of SPECT (single photon emission computed tomography) provides a three dimensional view of the myocardium with less overlap of structures. De Pasquale et al.[59] compared a visual and quantitative analysis of SPECT imaging in 291 patients and found a high sensitivity and specificity for the detection of pathology. Quantitative analysis involved the use of a bulls eye plot of maximum count circumferential profiles in the short axis view, and similar findings were reported by Maddahi et al.[60] using a polar display. SPECT stress redistribution imaging was found to be more accurate for the detection and extent of disease than planar imaging by Fintel et al.[61] and Maddahi et al.[62] in men but not in women where breast attenuation causes false positive defects. Quantification should take account of differences in mass of each slice. Prigent et al.[63] have described algorithms that rely on counts rather than edge detection which, in a dog model, was as accurate as estimates of slice weight. In clinical practice manual methods for measuring perfusion defects from vertical and long axis views, which are not as dependent on slice mass correction, have proved useful.[64]

An alternative approach to improving planar images that we have adopted in our laboratory is gating the thallium image to the electrocardiogram.[65] This provides a predictive accuracy of 91% in the detection of coronary artery disease and has the advantage of using a standard gamma camera, allowing acute imaging at the bedside. Three projections can be acquired in 15–20 minutes within the redistribution time of thallium-201 (myocardial uptake plateau 5–15 minutes)[66] and provide not only information about perfusion but also wall motion (Plate 8).

Alternatives to exercise

The stimulus to finding pharmacological challenge to replace exercise appears to have originated from the difficulties in dealing with motion artefacts during PET imaging. Gould et al.[67] have shown that incremental doses of dipyridamole cause increasing vasodilatation. Since then many studies have been reported showing similar sensitivities and specificities to exercise thallium studies,[68,69] especially with quantitative analysis.[70] In a recent study by Huikuri et al.[71] a protocol involving hand grip exercise following intravenous dipyridamole was found to be superior to bicycle exercise for the detection of multiple vessel disease using SPECT, probably due to the low workloads achieved during dynamic exercise. The preferred dose for intravenous use appears to be 0.56 mg/kg over four minutes[72] and this appears to be safe even in an elderly population (>70 years)[73] with chest pain occurring in 20–25% and aminophylline being required to reverse side effects in approximately 15%. More recently, oral dipyridamole in doses of 300–400 mg has been used in place of, or in addition to, a restricted exercise test[74] but imaging times, especially for reperfusion images, require to be prolonged due to the altered washout characteristics.[75]

The provocation of chest pain by dipyridamole has been suggested to be non-specific and unrelated to the extent of coronary artery disease[76] although it is difficult to reconcile this with the hypothesis that dipyridamole produces relative endocardial underperfusion. This does not appear to be the case with dipyridamole induced ST segment change, which occurs in 15–40% of patients. Two studies[77,78] have found that ST shift accurately identifies multiple vessel disease and particularly severe coronary disease >95% stenosis. Chambers et al.[79] found ST changes were related to the presence of 'good' collateral vessels and hypothesized that this may facilitate ischaemia or 'steal' with reduced distal flow in the collateral dependent vascular bed, particularly where the rate pressure product was increased with enhanced myocardial oxygen demand.

Diagnostic and prognostic value

Exercise thallium scintigraphy has an established place in the identification of patients with coronary artery disease[80,81] which is superior to exercise testing alone.[82] The addition of reperfusion imaging for the identification of epicardial scar[83] has similarly been widely accepted.

The addition of various quantitative approaches to the interpretation of images and the subsequent measurements of washout of thallium[84] and more recently quantitative SPECT stress/redistribution imaging[61,62] have all served to improve the detection and localization of myocardial ischaemia.

Probability analysis, employing Bayes theorem[85,86] has shown that the diagnostic information provided by any test is largely determined by the prevalence of disease within the population. For thallium scintigraphy this is of most value when the pre-test probability is intermediate[87] and should be borne in mind when financial considerations are made.

Ladenheim et al.[88] assessed 1659 patients with symptoms suggestive of coronary artery disease to evaluate the incremental prognostic power of clinical history, exercise testing and thallium perfusion scintigraphy for the risk of subsequent events (cardiac death, myocardial infarction, late coronary artery surgery) over one year. This allowed a stratification for individual patient risk from 2–22% with significant additional prognostic information being gained when non-invasive testing with exercise electrocardiography and thallium-201 scintigraphy were used in groups of patients with intermediate or high probability of disease. By identifying patients at low risk, the authors calculated a cost saving of 64%. This study reaffirms that patients with normal thallium scintigraphy, either with or without associated coronary artery disease, have a low cardiac event rate (approximately 0.5% per year).[89,90] Though to use this model, an individual physician should apply his own thresholds for acceptable risk and, of course, should consider the disease probability for his patient population. Kaul et al.[91] found that for ambulatory patients with chest pain, referred for cardiac catheterisation, followed for 4–8 years that the number of diseased vessels (luminal diameter >50% narrowing) was the most important predictor of future cardiac events, followed by the number of segments demonstrating redistribution on delayed thallium-201 images, except for non-fatal myocardial infarction, for which redistribution was the most important predictor. A combination of catheterisation data and exercise thallium test was superior to either test alone.

Gill et al.[92] demonstrated that increased lung thallium uptake, considered to be a marker of left ventricular dysfunction during exercise was the best predictor of cardiac events over five years. In another study by Kaul et al.[93] with a four to nine year follow-up, reported a similar prognostic value for quantitative lung/heart ratio of thallium uptake although this was not confirmed in the previously mentioned study by Kaul[91] due probably to visual interpretation.

The overall conclusions are that for the patient with chest pain quantitative thallium-201 scintigraphy, scintigraphic variables either alone or in combination with exercise data are powerful predictors of subsequent death, non-fatal myocardial infarction or coronary artery bypass surgery.[94]

Following acute myocardial infarction exercise thallium scanning is able to stratify patients into low and high risk groups. Gibson et al.[95] have shown that the presence of abnormal scintigraphy with multiple defects on redistribution and increased lung uptake carries a higher risk for subsequent cardiac events than either the number of diseased vessels or left ventricular ejection fraction at rest. The same group[96] showed that in patients with single vessel disease after an uncomplicated myocardial infarction, the presence of reversible stress thallium defects in the infarct zone accurately predicted late ischaemic events (severe angina and recurrent myocardial infarction). Similarly, Brown et al.[97] demonstrated that reversible defects in the infarct zone were the best markers of future events.

Early exercise testing at 72 hours after acute myocardial infarction in selected patients with an uncomplicated course has been found to be safe.[98] Of 14 patients with a positive exercise thallium test, four subsequently suffered an adverse clinical event (reinfarction, angina, or VT in hospital) whereas 40 patients with a negative exercise thallium result had no adverse events. As an alternative to stress imaging, dipyridamole thallium imaging has also shown to be effective in provoking ischaemia in the peri-infarct setting[99] with those patients with reversible perfusion defects being more at risk of developing post-infarct angina in the subsequent months.[100]

Assessment of intervention

As perfusion imaging is more effective than arteriography in identifying the functional impact of stenosis in patients with multiple vessel disease, imaging may provide a method of identifying the distribution of vessels which are primarily responsible for ischaemia. Briesblatt et al.[101] have used SPECT thallium imaging to identify the primary stenosis or 'culprit lesion' and performed percutaneous transluminal coronary angioplasty (PTCA) to this lesion. A second exercise test 2–4 weeks later divided the patients into two roughly equal groups. In those with no evidence of ischaemia in a second vascular territory, 13% required PTCA to a second vessel at one year, and a second group with further evidence of myocardial ischaemia 47% having further PTCA and 79% multi-vessel PTCA at one year. In 26 of these 38 patients in the second group the thallium defects were new, due presumably to unmasking of a second ischaemic area. The thallium scan appears to be an effective method of predicting future events and the need for further intervention. Miller et al.[102] looked at a number of clinical, angiographic and thallium variables and demonstrated that the post PTCA pressure gradient (>20 mmHg) predicted clinical events and treatment events (PTCA or coronary bypass surgery) and that the number of segments showing reversible thallium defects or slower thallium clearance predicted clinical events, treatment events and restenosis. The combination of angiographic (post PTCA gradient) and perfusion variables were additive predictors of adverse events at one year, the relative risk for this being four times greater in patients with these variables. Similar findings with respect to reversible thallium perfusion defects have been made with SPECT dipyridamole thallium imaging.[103] Data presented by Manyari et al.[104] suggests that following successful angioplasty with no clinical or angiographic evidence of restenosis, exercise induced scintigraphic abnormalities may take up to three months to resolve and the authors postulate 'mismatch' of perfusion with thallium uptake in these 'stunned' regions of myocardium. As suggested by Kiat and Berman[105] remodelling of the artery would certainly seem a more likely explanation and thallium scintigraphy early at 2–4 weeks post angioplasty would appear to be more appropriate for patient management (Plate 9).

Following coronary bypass surgery, several studies have shown the value of thallium perfusion scanning for assessing graft patency or progressive disease in the native vessels[106-108] especially with the addition of quantitative assessment with thallium washout rates.[109] Interestingly, careful analysis of 'persistent' defects prior to coronary artery bypass grafting has shown that roughly half are capable of improved perfusion, suggesting that thallium-201 'fixed' defects are compatible with not only scar tissue but also reversibly ischaemic myocardium.[110,111] A more recent study[112] has suggested that performing late redistribution images (18–72 hours) could effectively differentiate between segments that are viable and those that are essentially scar tissue.

Acute myocardial infarction

Work by F J Wackers[113] has amply demonstrated the value of thallium imaging, especially in the first six hours after the onset of symptoms, in localizing the site or with direct comparison of in vivo images and post mortem findings of the size of infarction.[114] Care has to be taken to differentiate between acutely ischaemic tissue, which is viable, in the patient presenting with unstable angina[115] and infarct. This usually requires a reperfusion scan[116] and an assessment of wall function, which can be obtained from a gated thallium image. Infarct sizing acutely[117] can provide valuable immediate information especially in patients with very extensive infarcts, in whom the prognosis is poor (Plate 10).

With the advent of thrombolytic therapy, thallium is increasingly being employed as the method of assessing efficacy of reperfusion.[118] The timing of the thallium administration is important: given either intracoronary or intravenously soon after reperfusion, images reflect hyperaemic flow rather than the extent of viable myocardium. When thallium is given prior to reperfusion, during the occlusive phase, redistribution images or rest images at 24 hours, more accurately reflect the degree of reperfusion. That the degree of improvement in the size of thallium defect is a measure of viable myocardium has been suggested by experimental studies using $[^{18}F]$-2-deoxyglucose uptake (FDG) (a positron emitter and tracer of exogenous glucose uptake).[119,120] Two recent studies,[121,122] again using PET imaging with FDG and $[^{13}N]$–ammonia but not in the acute setting of infarct, have suggested that thallium may underestimate the extent of viable myocardium. The combined use of metabolic and flow markers with PET imaging holds promise as the most accurate measure of viable myocardial tissue.

The development of technetium-99m labelled isonitrile compounds, as an alternative to thallium-201, show promise as tracers of myocardial perfusion. Of those used in humans, technetium-99m methoxy-isobutyl-isonitrile (Tc–MIBI) has the fastest hepatic clearance and least lung uptake resulting in good myocardial to background ratios, although myocardial extraction fraction is lower than thallium.[123,124] As Tc-MIBI does not redistribute, rest/stress protocols[125] have to be employed to demonstrate reversible ischaemia, but this feature makes it feasible to assess reperfusion and to employ the advantageous imaging characteristics of technetium with SPECT.

In summary, with the advent of thrombolytic therapy and the application of interventional techniques in the acute coronary syndromes, perfusion imaging has a valuable part to play in the assessment and timing of such interventions. It also provides unique, non-invasive data which can be of inestimable value in the assessment of the patient with chest pain and in the management of the patient with coronary heart disease.

REFERENCES

1 Marcus ML. The coronary collateral circulation. In: The coronary circulation in health and disease. New York: McGraw-Hill, 1983: p. 221

2 Marcus ML. Effects of cardiac hypertrophy on the coronary circulation in health and disease. In: The coronary circulation in health and disease. New York: McGraw-Hill, 1983: p. 285

3 Marcus ML. Physiological effects of a coronary stenosis. In: The coronary circulation in health and disease. New York: McGraw-Hill, 1983: p. 242

4 Ganz W, Tamura K, Marcus HF, Donoso R, Yoshida S, Swan HJC. Measurement of coronary sinus blood flow by continuous thermodilution in man. Circulation 1971; 44: 181

5 Marcus ML, Wilson RF, White CW. Methods of measurement of myocardial blood flow in patients: a critical review. Circulation 1987; 76: 245–253

6 Marcus ML, White CW, Kirchner PT. Isn't it time to reevaluate the sensitivity of noninvasive approaches for the diagnosis of coronary artery disease? J Am Coll Cardiol 1986; 8: 1033–1034

7 Harrison DC, White CW, Hiratzka LF et al. Can the significance of a coronary artery stenosis be predicted by quantitative coronary angiography. Circulation 1981; 64: 160–163

8 Marcus LM. The coronary circulation in health and disease. New York: McGraw-Hill 1983: p. 260

9 McPherson DD, Hiratzka LF, Lamber WC et al. Delineation of the extent of coronary atherosclerosis by high frequency echocardiography. N Engl J Med 1987; 316: 394–399

10 Glagov S, Weisenberg E, Zarins C, Stankunavicus R, Kolettis GJ. Compensatory enlargement of human atherosclerotic coronary arteries. N Engl J Med 1987; 316: 1371–1375

11 Beatt KJ, Luijten HE, de Feyter PJ, van den Brand M, Reiber JHC, Serruys PW. Change in diameter of coronary artery segments adjacent to stenosis after

percutaneous transluminal coronary angioplasty: Failure of percent diameter stenosis measurements to reflect morphologic changes induced by balloon dilatation. J Am Coll Cardiol 1988; 12: 315–323

12 Gould KL. Quantification of coronary stenosis in vivo. Circ Res 1985; 57: 341–353

13 Klocke FJ. Measurements of coronary blood flow and degree of stenosis: Current clinical implications and continuing uncertainties. J Am Coll Cardiol 1983; 1: 31

14 Gould KL. Assessing coronary stenosis severity – a recurrent clinical need. J Am Coll Cardiol 1986; 8: 91–94

15 Kirkeide RL, Gould KL, Parsel L. Assessment of coronary stenosis by myocardial perfusion imaging during pharmacological coronary vasodilation VII validation of coronary flow reserve as a single integrated functional measure of stenosis severity reflecting all its geometric dimensions. J Am Coll Cardiol 1986; 7: 103–113

16 Klocke FJ. Measurement of coronary flow reserve: defining pathophysiology versus making decisions about patient care. Circulation 1987; 76: 1183–1189

17 Hoffman JIE. A critical review of coronary reserve. Circulation 1987; 75: Part 2, i6–i11

18 Hoffman JIE. Coronary flow reserve. Current Opinion in Cardiology 1988; 3(suppl 6): 874–880

19 Rutishauser W, Simon H, Stacky JP, Schad N, Noseda G, Wellaner J. Evaluation of roentgen cinedensitometry for flow measurements in models and the intact circulation. Circulation 1967; 36: 951

20 Smith HC, Frye RI, Donald DE. Roetgen videodensitometric measurements of coronary blood flow. Determination from simultaneous indicator-dilution curves to selected sites in the coronary circulation and in coronary artery saphenous vein grafts. Mayo Clin Proc 1971; 46: 800

21 Vogel R, LeFrel M, Bates E, O'Neill W, Foster R, Kirlin P, Smith D, Pitt B. Application of digital techniques to selective coronary arteriography: use of myocardial contrast appearance time to measure coronary flow reserve. Am Heart J 1984; 107: 153

22 Mancini GBJ, Higgins CB. Digital subtraction angiography: a review of cardiac applications. Prog Cardiovasc Dis 1985; 18: 111

23 Wangler Rd, Peters KG, Laughlin DE, Tomasek RJ, Marcus ML. A method for continuously assessing coronary velocity in the rat. Am J Physiol 1981; 10: H816

24 Marcus M, Wright C, Doty D, Eastham C, Laughlin D, Krumm P, Fasteron C, Bray M. Measurement of coronary velocity and reactive hyperemia in the coronary circulation of humans. Circ Res 1981; 49: 877

25 White CW, Right CB, Doty DB et al. Does visual interpretation of the coronary arteriogram predict the physiological significance of a coronary stenosis. N Engl J Med 1984; 310: 819

26 Harrison D, Ferguson D, Collins S et al. Rethrombosis after reperfusion with streptokinase: importance of geometry of residual lesions. Circulation 1984; 69: 991

27 Wilson RF, White CW. Measurement of maximal coronary flow reserve: a technique for assessing the physiologic significance of coronary arterial lesions in humans. Herz 1987; 12: 163–176

28 Wilson RF, Marcus ML, White CU. Prediction of the physiologic significance of coronary arterial lesions by qualitative lesion geometry in patients with limited coronary artery disease. Circulation 1987; 75: 723

29 Ritchie JL, Hamilton GW, Gould KL, Allen D, Kennedy JW, Hammermeister KE. Myocardial imaging with [133m]indium and [99m]technetium -macro aggregated albumin. Am J Cardiol 1975; 35: 380–389

30 Phelps ME, Mazziotta JC, Schelbert HR. Positron emission tomography and

autoradiography. Principles and applications for the brain and heart. Vol 12, New York: Raven Press, 1986: p. 591

31 Selwyn AP, Shea MJ, Focle R et al. Regional myocardial and organ blood flow after myocardial infarction: application of the microsphere principle in man. Circulation 1986; 73: 433

32 Eckenhoff JE, Hafkenschiel JH, Harmer MH et al. Measurement of coronary blood flow by the nitrous oxide method. Am J Physiol 1948; 152: 356

33 Cibulski AA, Markov A, Lehan PH et al. External measurement and mapping of myocardial isotope after coronary venous [85]Krypton and [133]Xenon injections. Am J Cardiol 1974; 34: 545–551

34 Herd JA, Hollenberg M, Thronburn GD, Kopald HH, Barger AC. Myocardial blood flow determined with Krypton 85 in unanesthetised dogs. Am J Physiol 1962; 203: 122–124

35 Ross RS, Ueda K, Lichtlen PR, Rees JR. Measurement of myocardial blood flow in animals and man by selective injection of radioactive inert gas into the coronary arteries. Circ Res 1964; 15: 28–41

36 Kety SS. Theory and applications of exchange of inert gas at lungs and tissues. Pharmacol Rev 1951; 3: 1–41

37 Conn HL. Equilibrium distribution of radioxenon in tissue-Xenon-haemoglobin association curve. J Appl Physiol 1961; 16: 1065–1070

38 Cannon PI, Dell RB, Dwyer EM. Measurement of regional myocardial perfusion in man with 133-Xenon and a scintillation camera. J Clin Invest 1972; 51: 964–977

39 Parkey RW, Lewis SE, Stokely EM, Boute FJ. Compartmental analysis of the 133-Xenon regional myocardial blood flow curve. Radiology 1972; 104: 425–426

40 Holman BL, Adams DF, Jewitt D et al. Measuring regional myocardial blood flow with 133-Xenon and the Anger camera. Radiology 1974; 112: 99–107

41 Engel H-J, Heron R, Liese W, Hundeshagen H, Lichtlen P. Regional myocardial perfusion at rest in coronary disease assessed by microsphere scintigraphy and inert gas clearance. Am J Cardiol 1976; 37: 134

42 Maseri A, Mancini P, L'Abbate A, Magini G. Method for regional dynamic study of myocardial blood flow in man. J Nucl Biol Med 1971; 15: 54–57

43 Engel H-J. Assessment of regional myocardial blood flow by the precordial 133-Xenon clearance technique. In: The Pathophysiology of Myocardial Perfusion, 1979: p. 60

44 Maseri A, L'Abbate A, Michelassi C et al. Possibilities, limitations and technique for the study of regional myocardial perfusion in man by Xenon-133. Cardiovasc Res 1977; 11: 277–290

45 Hirzel HO, Krayenbuehl. Validity of the 133-Xenon method for measuring coronary blood flow. Comparison with coronary sinus outflow determined by an electromagnetic flow probe. Pflugers Arch 1974; 349: 159–169

46 McIntyre WJ, Cannon PJ, Ashburn WL. Measurements of regional myocardial perfusion. In: Pierson RH, Kriss JP, Jones RH, McIntyre WJ, eds. Quantitative Nuclear Cardiology. New York: Wiley, 1975: pp. 57–67

47 Smith SC, Gorlin R, Herman MV, Taylor WJ, Collin JJ. Myocardial blood flow in man – Effects of coronary collateral circulation and coronary artery bypass surgery. J Clin Invest 1972; 51: 2556–2565

48 Zierler KL. Equation for measuring blood flow by external monitoring of radioisotopes. Circ Res 1965; 16: 309–321

49 L'Abbate A, Maseri A. Xenon studies of myocardial blood flow: theoretical, technical and practical aspects. Semin Nucl Med 1980; X, 1: 2–15

50 Martin W, Tweddel AC, McGhie I, Hutton I. Coronary flow response to stress in normal coronary arteries. Eur J Nucl Med 1987; 1: 119–125

51 Asokar SK, Fraser RL, Kolbeck RL, Frank MJ. Variations in right and left

coronary blood flow in man with and without occlusive coronary disease. Br Heart J 1975; 37: 604

52 Klocke FJ. Measurements of coronary blood flow and degree of stenosis: Current clinical implications and continuing uncertainties. J Am Coll Cardiol 1983; 1: 31–41

53 Smith SC, Gorlin R, Herman MV, Taylor WJ, Collin JJ. Myocardial blood flow in man – effects of coronary collateral circulation and coronary artery bypass surgery. J Clin Invest 1972; 51: 2556–2565

54 Hutchins GM, Bulkley BH, Ridolfi RL, Griffith LSC, Lohr ET, Piaso MA. Correlation of coronary arteriograms and left ventriculograms with post mortem studies. Circulation 1976; 54: 162

55 Ideker R, Behar V, Starr J et al. Evaluation of asynergy as an indicator of myocardial fibrosis. Circulation 1976; 54: 40

56 Rentrop P, Cohen M, Blarke H, Philips R. Changes in collateral channel filling immediately after controlled coronary artery occlusion by an angioplasty balloon in human subjects. J Am Coll Cardiol 1985; 5: 587

57 Matsuda Y, Ogawa H, Moritoni K et al. Transient appearance of collaterals during vasospastic occlusion in patients without obstructive coronary atherosclerosis. Am Heart J 1985; 4: 759

58 Tweddel AC. Relations between coronary perfusion and myocardial function. L'information Cardiologique 1987; XI: 111–114

59 De Pasquale EE, Nody AC, De Puey EG et al. Quantitative rotational thallium 201 tomography for identifying and localising coronary artery disease. Circ 1988; 7: 316–327

60 Maddahi J, Abdulla A, Garcia EV, Swan HJ, Berman DS. Noninvasive identification of left main and triple vessel coronary artery disease: improved accuracy using quantitative analysis of regional myocardial stress distribution and washout of thallium-201. J Am Coll Cardiol 1986; 7: 22A

61 Fintel DJ, Links JM, Brinker JA, Frank TL, Parker M, Becker L. Improved diagnostic performance of exercise thallium-201 single photon emission computed tomography over planar imaging in the diagnosis of coronary artery disease. J Am Coll Cardiol (In press)

62 Maddahi J, Van Train KF, Wong C et al. Comparison of T1-201 single photon emission computerised tomography (SPECT) and planar imaging for evaluation of coronary artery disease. J Nucl Med 1986; 27: 999

63 Prigent F, Maddahi J, Garcia EV, Risser K, Lew AS, Berman DS. Comparative methods for quantifying myocardial infarct size by thallium 201 SPECT. J Nucl Med 1987; 28: 325–333

64 Maublast JC, Peycelon P, Cardot JC, Verderet JV, Fagret D, Comet M. Value of myocardial defect size measured by thallium-201 SPECT: Results of a multicentre trial comparing heparin and a new fibrinolytic agent. J Nucl Med 1988; 29: 1486–1491

65 Martin W, Tweddel AC, McGhie AI, Hutton I. Gated thallium scintigraphy in patients with coronary artery disease. Clin Phys Physiol Meas 1987; 8: 343–354

66 Chervu LR. Radiopharmaceuticals in cardiovascular nuclear medicine. Semin Nucl Med 1979; IX, 4: 241–256

67 Gould KL. Non-invasive assessment of coronary stenoses by myocardial imaging during pharmacologic coronary vasodilatation. II. Clinical methodology and feasibility. Am J Cardiol 1978; 41: 279

68 Ruddy TD, Dighero HR, Newell JB et al. Quantitative analysis of dipyridamole-thallium images for the detection of coronary artery disease. J Am Coll Cardiol 1987; 10: 142–149

69 Josephson MA, Brown GB, Hecht HS et al. Noninvasive detection and localisation of coronary stenoses in patients: comparison of resting dipyridamole and exercise thallium-201 myocardial perfusion imaging. Am Heart J 1982; 103: 1008–1018

70 Demongart JL, Constantinesco A, Mossard JM et al. Evaluation of myocardial perfusion and left ventricular function by thallium scintigraphy after dipyridamole. Eur J Nucl Med 1981; 6: 491–503

71 Huikuri H, Kohronen VR, Airaksine KEJ, Ikaheimo MJ, Heikkila J, Takkunen JT. Comparison of dipyridamole handgrip test and bicycle exercise test for thallium tomographic imaging. Am J Cardiol 1988; 61: 264–268

72 Iskandrian AS, Heo J, Askerase A et al. Dipyridamole cardiac imaging. Am Heart J 1988; 115: 432–443

73 Lam JYT, Chaitman BR, Glaenzer M. Safety and diagnostic accuracy of dipyridamole-thallium in the elderly. J Am Coll Cardiol 1988; 11,3: 585–589

74 Wilde P, Walker P, Watt I, Reese JR, Davies ER. Thallium myocardial imaging: Recent experience using coronary vasodilation. Clin Radiol 1982; 33: 43–50

75 Ruddy TD, Gill JB, Finkelstein DM. Myocardial uptake and clearance of thallium 201 in normal subjects: comparison of dipyridamole induced hyperemia with exercise stress. J Am Coll Cardiol 1987; 10: 547–556

76 Pearlman JD, Boucher CA. Diagnostic value for coronary artery disease of chest pain during dipyridamole-thallium stress testing. Am J Cardiol 1988; 61: 43–45

77 Essandoh LK, Iapeyre AC, Gibbons RJ. The significance of ECG changes during dipyridamole thallium-201 myocardial scintigraphy. J Nucl Med 1988; 29: 945

78 Reisman S, Klepser C, Vaugeois JC, Sacchi T, Konka S. ST segment depression during intravenous dipyridamole thallium infusion: identification of patients with extensive jeopardized myocardium. J Nucl Med 1988; 29: 782

79 Chambers CE, Brown KA. Dipyridamole-induced ST segment depression during thallium-201 imaging in patients with coronary artery disease: angiographic and hemodynamic determinants. J Am Coll Cardiol 1988; 12: 37–41

80 Bailey IK, Griffith LSC, Roulea J, Strauss W, Pitt B. Thallium-201 myocardial perfusion imaging at rest and during exercise. Circ 1977; 55: 79–87

81 Ritchie JL, Trobaugh GB, Hamilton GW, Gould KL, Narahana KA, Murray JA, Williams DL. Myocardial imaging with thallium-201 at rest and during exercise. Circ 1977; 56: 66–713

82 Botvinick EH, Taradash MR, Shames DM, Parmley WM. Thallium-201 myocardial perfusion scintigraphy for the clinical classicication of normal, abnormal and equivocal electrocardiographic stress tests. Am J Cardiol 1978; 41: 43

83 Leppo J, Yipintsoi T, Blankstein R et al. Thallium 201 myocardial scintigraphy in patients with triple vessel disease and ischemic exercise stress tests. Circ 1979; 59: 714–721

84 Garcia EV, Van Train K, Maddahi J et al. Quantification of rotational thallium 201 myocardial tomography. J Nucl Med 1985; 26: 17–26

85 Diamond GA, Forrester JS. Analysis of probability as an aid in the clinical diagnosis of coronary artery disease. N Engl J Med 1979; 300: 1350–1358

86 Melin JA, Piret LJ, Vasbutsele RMJ et al. Diagnostic value of exercise electrocardiography and thallium myocardial scintigraphy in patients without previous myocardial infarction: A Bayesian Approach. Circ 1981; 63: 1019–1024

87 Murray RG, McKillop JH, Bessent RG, Lorimer AR, Hutton I, Lawrie TDV. Bayesian analysis of stress thallium-201 scintigraphy. Eur J Nucl Med 1981; 6: 201

88 Ladenheim ML, Kotler TS, Pollock BH, Berman DS, Diamond GA. Incremental prognostic powers of clinical history, exercise electrocardiography and myocardial perfusion scintigraphy in suspected coronary artery disease. Am J Cardiol 1987; 59: 270–277

89 Wackers FJ, Russo DS, Russo D, Clements JP. Prognostic significance of

normal quantitative planar thallium-201 stress scintigraphy in patients with chest pain. J Am Coll Cardiol 1985; 6: 27–30

90 Brown KA, Boucher CA, Okada RD et al. Prognostic value of exercise thallium 201 imaging in patients presenting for evaluation of chest pain. J Am Coll Cardiol 1983; 1: 994–1001

91 Kaul S, Lilly DR, Gascho JA et al. Prognostic utility of the exercise thallium-201 test in ambulatory patients with chest pain: comparison with cardiac catheterisation. Circ 1988; 77: 745–758

92 Gill JB, Ruddy TD, Newell JB, Finkelstein DM, Strauss HW, Boucher CA. Prognostic importance of thallium uptake by the lungs during exercise in coronary artery disease. N Engl J Med 1987; 317: 1485–1489

93 Kaul S, Finkelstein DM, Homnia S, Leavitt M, Okada RD, Boucher CA. Superiority of quantitative exercise thallium-201 variables in determining long-term prognosis in ambulatory patients with chest pain: a comparison with cardiac catheterisation. J Am Coll Cardiol 1988; 12: 25–34

94 Cerqueira M, Ritchie JL. Thallium 201 scintigraphy in risk assessment for ambulatory patients with chest pain: does everyone need catheterisation? J Am Coll Cardiol 1988; 12: 35–36

95 Gibson RS, Watson DD, Craddock GB et al. Prediction of cardiac events after uncomplicated myocardial infarction: a prospective study comparing predischarge exercise thallium-201 scintigraphy and coronary angiography. Circ 1983; 68: 321–336

96 Wilson WW, Gibson RS, Nygaard TW et al. Acute myocardial infarction associated with single vessel coronary artery disease: an analysis of clinical outcome and the prognostic importance of vessel patency and residual ischemic myocardium. J Am Coll Cardiol 1988; 11: 223–234

97 Brown KA, Weiss RM, Clements JP, Wackers FJTh. Usefulness of residual ischemic myocardium within prior infarct zone for identifying patients at high risk late after acute myocardial infarction. Am J Cardiol 1987; 60: 15–19

98 Topol EJ, Jain JE, O'Neill WW, Nicklas JM, Shea MJ, Burek K, Pitt B. Exercise testing three days after onset of acute myocardial infarction. Am J Cardiol 1987; 60: 958–962

99 Leppo J, O'Brien J, Rothendler JA, Getchell JD, Lee VW. Dipyridamole thallium-201 scintigraphy in the prediction of future cardiac events after myocardial infarction. N Engl J Med 1984; 310: 1014–1018

100 Pirelli S, Inglese E, Suppa M, Corrada E, Campolo L. Dipyridamole-thallium 201 scintigraphy in the early post-infarction period (Safety and accuracy in predicting the extent of coronary disease and future recurrence of angina in patients suffering from their first myocardial infarction). Eur Heart J 1988; 9: 1324–1331

101 Briesblatt WM, Barnes JV, Weland F, Spaccoverto LJ. Incomplete revascularisation in multivessel percutaneous transluminal coronary angioplasty: The role for stress thallium-201 imaging. J Am Coll Cardiol 1988; 11: 1183–1190

102 Miller D, Lui P, Strauss W, Block PC, Okada RD, Boucher CA. Prognostic value of computer-quantitated exercise thallium imaging early after percutaneous transluminary coronary angioplasty. J Am Coll Cardiol 1987; 10: 275–283

103 Jain A, Mahmaria JJ, Borges-Neto S et al. Clinical significance of perfusion defects by thallium 201 single photon emission tomography following oral dipyridamole early after coronary angioplasty. J Am Coll Cardiol 1988; 11: 970–976

104 Manyari DE, Knudtson M, Kloiber R, Roth D. Sequential thallium 201 myocardial perfusion studies after successful percutaneous transluminal coronary artery angioplasty: delayed resolution of exercise-induced scintigraphic abnormalities. Circ 1988; 77: 86–95

105 Kiat H, Berman DS. Scintigraphic assessment of myocardial viability and perfusion. Curr Opinion Cardiol 1988; 3: 922–936

106 Wainwright RJ, Bresnand-Roper DA, Maisey MN, Sowton E. Exercise thallium 201 myocardial scintigraphy in the follow up of aortocoronary bypass graft surgery. Br Heart J 1980; 43: 56–66

107 Pfisterer M, Emmenegger H, Schmitt et al. Accuracy of serial myocardial perfusion scintigraphy with thallium-201 for prediction of graft patency early and late after coronary bypass surgery. A controlled prospective study. Circ 1982; 66: 1017–1024

108 Kolibash AJ, Call TD, Bush CA, Tetalman MR, Lewis RP. Myocardial perfusion as an indicator of graft patency after coronary artery bypass surgery. Circ 1980; 61: 882–887

109 Zimmermann R, Tillmanns H, Knapp WH, Neumann F-J, Saggau W, Kubler W. Noninvasive assessment of coronary artery bypass patency: Determination of myocardial thallium-201 washout rates. Eur Heart J 1988; 9: 319–327

110 Lui P, Kiess MC, Okada RD et al. The persistent defect on exercise thallium imaging and its fate after myocardial revascularisation: does it represent scar or ischemia? Am Heart J 1985; 110: 996–1001

111 Fioretti P, Reijs AEM, Neumann D et al. Improvement in transient and 'persistent' perfusion defects on early and late post-exercise thallium-201 tomograms after coronary artery bypass grafting. Eur Heart J 1988; 9(12): 1332–1338

112 Kiat H, Berman D, Maddahi J, Yang LD, Van Train K. Late reversibility of tomographic myocardial thallium-201 defects: an accurate marker of myocardial viability. J Am Coll Cardiol 1988; 12: 1456–1463

113 Wackers FJTh, Busemann Sokole E, Samson G, Vd Schoot JB, Lie KI, Liem KL, Wellens HJJ. Value and limitation of thallium-201 scintigraphy in the acute phase of myocardial infarction. N Engl J Med 1976; 295: 1

114 Wackers FJTh, Becker AE, Samson G, Busemann Sokole E, Vd Schoot JB, Vet AJTM, Lie KI, Durrer D, Wellens H. Location and size of acute transmural myocardial infarction estimated from thallium-201 scintiscans. Circ 1977; 56,1: 72–78

115 Brown KA, Okada RD, Boucher CA, Phillips HR, Strauss HW, Pohost GM. Serial thallium-201 imaging at rest in patients with unstable and stable angina pectoris: relationship of myocardial perfusion at rest to presenting clinical symptoms. Am Heart J 1983; 106: 70–71

116 Wackers FJTh. Thallium-201 myocardial scintigraphy in acute myocardial infarction and ischemia. Seminars in Nuclear Medicine 1980; X,2: 127–144

117 Tweddel AC, Martin W, McGhie I, Hutton I. Infarct size can be measured acutely in developing myocardial infarction. Br Heart J 1988; 2: 29

118 Beller GA. Role of myocardial perfusion imaging in evaluating thrombolytic therapy for acute myocardial infarction. J Am Coll Cardiol 1987; 9: 661–668

119 Sochor H, Schwaiger M, Schelbert HR et al. Relationship between T1–201, Tc99m (sn) pryophosphate and F-18 2-deoxyglucose uptake in ischaemically injured dog myocardium. Am Heart J 1987; 114: 1066–1077

120 Melin JA, Wijns W, Keyeux A et al. Assessment of thallium-201 redistribution versus glucose uptake as predictors of viability after coronary occlusion and reperfusion. Circ 1988; 77: 927–934

121 Brunkes R, Schwaiger M, Grover-McKay M, Phelps ME, Tillisch J, Schelbert HR. Positron emission tomography detects tissue metabolic activity in myocardial segments with persistent thallium perfusion defects. J Am Coll Cardiol 1987; 10: 557–567

122 Tamaki N, Yonekura Y, Senda M et al. Value and limitation of stress thallium-201 single photon emission computed tomography: comparison with nitrogen-13-ammonia positron tomography. J Nucl Med 1988; 29: 1181–1188

123 Sia STB, Holman BC. Dynamic myocardial imaging in ischemic heart disease: use of technetium-99m isonitriles. Am J Card Imaging 1987; 1: 125–131

124 Stiner H, Buell U, Kleinhaus E, Bares R, Grosse W. Myocardial kinetics of 99Tc hexiakis-(2-methoxy-isobutyl-isonitrile) (HMIBI) in patients with coronary heart disease: a comparative study versus 201-T1 and SPECT. Nucl Med Commun 1988; 9: 15–23

125 Taillefer R, Laflamme L, Duprae G, Pickard M, Phareuf DC, Leveille J. Myocardial perfusion imaging with ^{99m}Tc-methoxy-isobutyl-isonitrile (MIBI): comparison of short and long time intervals between rest and stress injections preliminary results. Eur J Nucl Med 1988; 13: 515–522

British Medical Bulletin (1989) Vol. 45, No. 4, pp. 922–932

Whole heart distribution of myocardial perfusion, metabolism and myocardial viability by positron emission tomography

L I Araujo
A Maseri
Royal Postgraduate Medical School, Hammersmith Hospital, London, UK

The three dimensional evaluation of regional myocardial perfusion and metabolism of the whole left ventricular wall is now possible using the new generation of Positron Emission Tomography scanners (PET). We have used whole heart PET to study the metabolic consequences of transient myocardial ischaemia distal to critical coronary obstructions and to assess the viability of non contractile myocardium.

At present whole heart PET should be considered a sophisticated technique for clinical research but its remarkable potential and further possible technical advances suggest its diagnostic application could be considered in the future, if justified on a cost benefit basis.

Coronary blood is controlled by numerous factors and rapidly responds to changes in myocardial demand as a consequence of changes in cardiac work. This equilibrium is altered when coronary artery disease occurs and coronary blood flow becomes

0007–1420/89/0045–0922/$10.00

inadequate to match myocardial demand either because blood flow cannot increase as myocardial work increases or because of a primary reduction in flow with no change in myocardial demand. This imbalance between coronary blood flow and myocardial demand leads to a change in myocardial oxygen and substrate delivery and utilization causing immediate metabolic and mechanical abnormalities.

The possibility of assessing regional myocardial blood flow and metabolism at rest, during physiological and pharmacological interventions would allow the direct assessment of the adequacy of myocardial perfusion, oxygen and substrate delivery and utilization.

Whole heart Positron Emission Tomography (PET) offers the possibility of assessing regional myocardial perfusion and metabolism in man non-invasively and of establishing direct correlations with coronary artery anatomy and with ventricular function over the entire left ventricle. After a brief description of the technical aspects of PET, this overview will discuss the insights into pathophysiology of ischaemic heart disease obtained by determining regional abnormalities of glucose uptake caused by ischaemia and myocardial viability in akinetic zones of the left ventricular wall.

TECHNICAL CONSIDERATIONS

Positron emission tomography involves the use of short lived positron emitting isotopes such as ^{15}O, ^{13}N, ^{82}Rb, ^{81}Rb, ^{18}F that can label physiological substances such as ^{15}O-water, $[^{11}C]$-glucose or analogues such as $[^{18}F]$-deoxyglucose. Compared with the much more widely used single photon emitting tracers, such as thallium-201 and technitium-99m, positron emitting tracers offer the advantage of a much more accurate 3D reconstruction of the tracer distribution within the body and furthermore they allow precise regional quantification of the tracer concentration within the body.

A positron emitted from the nucleus during the radioactive decay process, travels few millimetres in tissue and when it interacts with an electron it produces simultaneously, two 511 keV gamma rays travelling in opposite directions. Thus, at an angle of 180 degrees sets of detectors placed at opposite sides of the body, can record in coincidence the simultaneous emission of gamma rays from the same positron. This mode of data collection offers a number of advantages compared with conventional single photon detection techniques such as attenuation correction, uniform resolution and uniform sensitivity[1] which allow the precise quantification of the regional tracer concentration within the body.

The present scanners consist of a circular array of 4000 detectors around the body which gives fifteen cross-sectional images of the heart simultaneously, each 7mm in thickness, over a field of view of 10.5 cm. The myocardial tracer distribution can be measured accurately and reconstructed tomographically in any desired orientation or as a complete 3D image of the heart in any desired projection.

MEASUREMENT OF REGIONAL MYOCARDIAL PERFUSION

A method has been developed for the quantification of regional myocardial blood flow based on the myocardial uptake and washout of ^{15}O water ($H_2^{15}O$) during a 3 minute inhalation of $C^{15}O_2$ (which is immediately transformed to $H_2^{15}O$ by carbonic anhydrase in the blood).

This technique has been validated in dogs versus the standard microsphere technique over a range of flow from 0.4 to 6ml/min/g of myocardium with a correlation coefficient of $r = 0.97$ ($P < 0.05$) not significantly different from the identity line.

ASSESSMENT OF TRANSIENT MYOCARDIAL ISCHAEMIA

Major metabolic changes during ischaemia

The aerobic myocardium preferentially uses free fatty acids for producing energy. However, during hypoxia or ischaemia, glucose becomes the most important substrate to maintain energy production. This switchover is due to a number of alterations of key regulatory steps in the intermediate metabolism. Reduced oxygen availability slows the electron transport chain in the mitochondria and leads to a rapid decrease in the rate of free fatty acid oxidation which in turn are accumulated in the cytosol as triglycerides. On the other hand glucose supply is increased by an increment of glycogen breakdown and increased uptake of exogenous glucose.

Although the rate of anaerobic glycolysis is enhanced under these circumstances, the progressive accumulation of H^+ ions will inhibit the enzymatic activity of key regulatory steps which in turn will reduce the rate of glucose utilization with the consequent reduction of energy production necessary for the cellular physiological processes.[2,3] If oxygen supply is re-established before irreversible cellular damage has occurred, glucose utilization remains enhanced, and free fatty acid oxidation decreased.

This pathophysiological information, obtained from different animal models of hypoxia and ischaemia, provided the rationale for studying myocardial glucose metabolism in patients after transient ischaemic episodes.

PET represents a suitable tool for the measurement of the regional uptake of glucose, or of its analogue deoxyglucose, in the areas of the myocardium which were caused to switch to glycolytic metabolism by ischaemia.

Previous studies with PET

Based on the observations in experimental animals, Camici and coworkers studied 12 patients with coronary artery disease and chronic stable angina using rubidium-82 (^{82}Rb) and [^{18}F]-deoxyglucose (FDG) to assess myocardial blood flow and exogenous glucose utilization.[4] The study revealed transient segmental defects of myocardial perfusion as indicated by ^{82}Rb defects during exercise testing, which caused angina and electrocardiographic signs of acute ischaemia. This regional perfusion abnormality disappeared 5 to 14 min after the end of the exercise. Myocardial glucose utilization, assessed after signs of acute ischaemia subsided by measuring FDG uptake, was increased in those myocardial areas which exhibited perfusion defects during exercise (Fig. 1). These findings are consistent with a slow and delayed metabolic recovery after a transient ischaemic episode.

Araujo and coworkers have employed the same tracers to assess myocardial perfusion and glucose metabolism in patients with unstable angina who had no clinical, electrocardiographic or enzymatic evidences of myocardial necrosis.[5] Twenty two patients were studied at rest and with no clinical or ECG evidence of acute myocardial ischaemia at the time of the study. Perfusion scans showed no regional defects of flow at rest; however, a significantly increased FDG uptake suggested an augmented myocardial exogenous glucose utilization despite the absence of recent episodes of

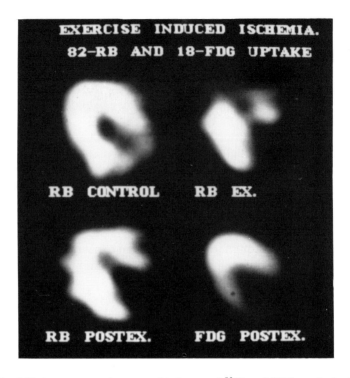

Fig. 1 Positron computed tomographic images of [82]Rb and FDG uptake in the same cross-sectional myocardial slice of a patient with severe LAD coronary stenosis. The [82]Rb scan at rest (top left) shows a uniform cation uptake in the wall of the left ventricle. A large apical and septal region becomes acutely ischemic during exercise, as shown by large defects on the [82]Rb scan recorded during the exercise test (top right). The [82]Rb scan recorded 6 min after the end of the exercise (bottom left) is comparable to the control. FDG was injected 9 min after the end of the exercise when all the signs of ischemia had reversed. The FDG scan (bottom right), recorded 60 min after tracer injection, outlines the previously ischemic area.

detectable acute ischaemia during scanning. These data indicate prolonged metabolic derangement of the myocardium of these patients, probably in connection with repetitive ischaemic episodes at rest characteristic of this syndrome. This metabolic pattern differed from that observed in normal volunteers and patients with chronic stable angina when studied under the same circumstances whereby the glucose utilization was found too low and homogeneous, which is typical of the normal fasting condition (Fig. 2). Other studies in patients with coronary disease and chronic stable angina indicate an inadequate response in free

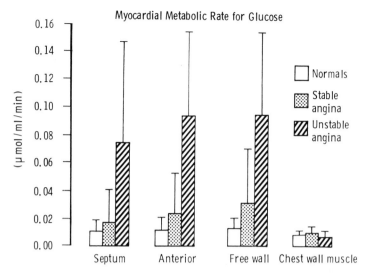

Fig. 2 This graph shows results of regional myocardial and chest muscle metabolic rate for glucose in normal volunteers (N), patients with stable angina (SA) and patients with unstable angina (UA). Glucose utilization was found to be increased in patients with UA as compared to both N and SA ($P < 0.001$ and $P < 0.01$, respectively). It should be noted that this increase in glucose utilization was confined to the myocardium as the chest wall muscle was similar in all three groups.

fatty acid utilization to increases of heart rate by atrial pacing.[6] These studies indicate that the free fatty acid oxidation remains attenuated in those areas supplied by stenotic arteries as compared with those regions supplied by normal arteries where an increased free fatty acid uptake proportion rate to the increase in myocardial contractile activity was found. These findings are consistent with the increased myocardial glucose utilization described above.

Studies in progress

New approaches to assess myocardial metabolism are under study in our institution with the latest generation of multiple slice positron scanners. This instrumentation brings about not only a much greater spatial resolution (6 mm compared to 16 mm of the previous scanner) but also the possibility of scanning the whole heart simultaneously in multiple slices which reveals anatomical details not available with previous systems. Studies to investigate myocardial metabolic changes associated with impaired coronary flow reserve are in progress.[7] Patients with chronic stable angina and single coronary artery disease were assessed at rest and after the intravenous infusion of dipyridamole which is a pharmacological test known to cause subendocardial ischaemia distal to critical coronary artery obstructions. Regional myocardial glucose utilization was measured after the test and compared with regional left ventricular mechanical function assessed by 2-D-echocardiography during the test. After the dipyridamole infusion increase of localized glucose uptake was present in those areas of myocardium supplied by stenosed arteries after the dipyridamole infusion (Fig. 3A–C). This metabolic abnormality was also seen in the absence of clinical and echocardiographic signs of myocardial

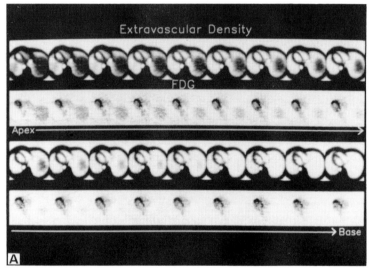

Fig. 3A This figure shows a typical example of increased regional myocardial [18F]-deoxyglucose (FDG) uptake in a patient with chronic stable angina and single vessel coronary disease which outlines the extension of the area which became ischaemic during the dipyridamole test. Two types of transaxial images of the heart are shown, on the top row the transmission scan from which the intravascular component has been subtracted (extra-vascular density) and immediately below the matching FDG image. Images have been recorded simultaneously from the apex to the base of the heart. In the territory of distribution of the obstructed left anterior descending artery, a marked uptake of FDG injected 20 min after the dipyridamole test can be seen. The distribution of FDG, extending towards the cavity of the left ventricle, is consistent with subendocardial distribution of myocardial ischaemia.

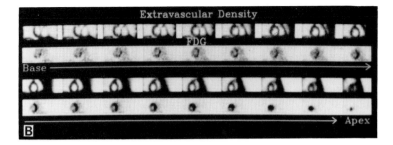

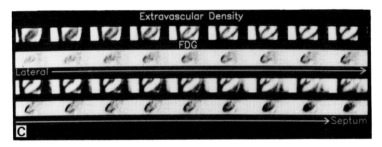

Fig. 3B, C This figure shows the same study but images have been reconstructed in a way to obtain slices perpendicular (B) and parallel (C) to the long axis of the left ventricle. Note the selective FDG myocardial uptake in the septum and anterior wall of the left ventricle.

ischaemia but occurred in the zones of the myocardium which had the lowest increase of regional coronary flow during the dipyridamole test. Our findings suggest that changes in substrate utilization can be detected earlier than other classical signs of acute ischaemia.

METABOLIC IMAGING AS A PREDICTOR OF MYOCARDIAL VIABILITY

The availability of procedures which can reperfuse ischaemic myocardium in a relative large number of patients brought about the need of identifying myocardial tissue with poor contractile function which could be potentially reversed by adequate revascularization. Indeed in some patients dramatic improvement in global ejection fraction and regional wall motion was observed after revascularization surgery. This improvement implies the presence of viable myocardium which before surgery had a chronic impairment of contractile function that was reversed by restoration of blood flow. This 'hibernating myocardium'[8] may result from either chronically reduced blood flow resulting in prolonged impairment of contractile function or from reduced contractile function leading to a reduction in oxygen consumption minimizing energy requirements caused by intermittent ischaemic episodes.

Prolonged but reversible mechanical abnormality has been observed after a period of coronary occlusion followed by complete reperfusion in animals and termed 'stunned myocardium'.[9]

Previous studies

Tillish and colleagues used PET in a group of patients who underwent revascularization surgery in an attempt to predict whether preoperative abnormalities in left ventricular wall motion were reversible.[10] Abnormalities of wall motion were assessed by either contrast or radionuclide angiography pre and post surgery. PET studies have been obtained before surgery using [13N]-ammonia as a flow marker and [18F]-deoxyglucose as a glucose metabolism tracer. Abnormal wall motion regions in which PET imaging showed preserved glucose uptake were predicted to be reversible whereas abnormal wall motion regions with decreased glucose uptake were predicted to be irreversible. The combined flow and metabolic imaging predicted reversible abnormalities with 85% accuracy and irreversible abnormalities with 92% accuracy.

Employing a similar approach to measure flow and glucose metabolism, Brunken and colleagues have studied patients with chronic infarction to assess whether there was viable tissue in those areas with electrocardiographic Q waves (11). PET showed that 54% of the Q wave regions had preserved glucose uptake suggesting the presence of substantial amount of viable tissue intermixed with scar and potentially salvageable.

STUDIES IN PROGRESS

We are pursuing an alternative method for assessing myocardial cell viability based on the measurement of rubidium-81 uptake at one hour after its intravenous injection. At this stage, the distribution of this tracer of potassium tends to be proportional to tissue potassium distribution in the organs and tissues which have a sufficiently rapid exchange with blood. Ischaemic myocardium having a flow of only 25% of normally perfused myocardium should reach 90% of equilibrium within 1 hour.

Thus the comparison of regional distribution of a flow indicator, $H_2{}^{15}O$, with that of ^{81}Rb can demonstrate areas of viable myocardium which take up ^{81}Rb, but receive inadequate myocardial perfusion.

CONCLUSIONS

Quantitative imaging of myocardial flow metabolism and tissue viability represents a novel method for evaluating the extent and severity of the myocardial ischaemic injury and for assessing contractile but viable myocardium. PET is an extremely sophisticated and costly technique which is now used to: (1) gain understanding of human pathophysiology; (2) assess the effect of therapeutic interventions; (3) establish correlations with other widely available techniques.

In the future the remarkable potential of this technique for assessing functional cardiac alteration may become of clinical use if justified on a cost/benefit basis.

REFERENCES

1 Lammertsma A, Frackowiak R. Positron emission tomography. CRC Crit Rev Biomed Eng 1987; 13: No. 2

2 Liedtke AJ. Alterations of carbohydrate and lipid metabolism in the acutely ischemic heart. Prog Cardiovasc Dis 1981; 23: 321–336

3 Taegtmeyer H. Myocardial metabolism. In: Phelps M, Mazziotta J, Schelbert H, eds. Positron Emission Tomography and Autoradiography: Principles and Applications for the Brain and Heart. New York: Raven Press, 1986: pp. 149–195

4 Camici P, Araujo LI, Spink T et al. Increased uptake of [^{18}F]-fluorodeoxyglucose in postischaemic myocardium of patients with exercise-induced angina. Circulation 1986; 74: 81–88

5 Araujo LI, Camici P, Spinks TJ, Jones T, Maseri A. Abnormalities in myocardial metabolism in patients with unstable angina as assessed by Positron Emission Tomography. Cardiovasc Drugs Ther 1988; 2: 41–46

6 Araujo LI, McFalls EO et al. Identification of Transient Regional Myocardial Metabolic Abnormalities in Patients with Chronic Stable Angina using Positron Emission Tomography. J Am Coll Cardiol 1989; 13: 45A

7 Grover-McKay M, Schelbert HR, Schwaiger M et al. Identification of impaired metabolic reserve by atrial pacing in patients with significant coronary artery stenosis. Circulation 1986; 74: 281–292

8 Braunwald E, Kloner RA. The stunned myocardium: Prolonged, postischemic ventricular dysfunction. Circulation 1982; 66: 1146–1149

9 Rahimtoola SH. A perspective on the three large multicenter randomized clinical trials of coronary bypass surgery for chronic stable angina. Circulation 1985; 8: V-123–V-135

10 Tillish J, Brunken R et al. Reversibility of Cardiac Wall Motion Abnormalities Presidented by Positron Tomography. N Engl J Med 1986; 314: 884–888
11 Brunken R, Tillisch J, Schwaiger M et al. Regional perfusion, glucose metabolism, and wall motion in patients with chronic electrocardiographic Q wave infarctions: evidence for persistence of viable tissue in some infarct regions by positron emission tomography. Circulation 1986; 73: No. 5

British Medical Bulletin (1989) Vol. 45, No. 4, pp. 933–947
© The British Council 1989

Cardiac magnetic resonance imaging

Anatomical display using spin echo images

S Rees
National Heart and Chest Hospitals, London, UK.

Magnetic resonance is a new method of imaging which is completely non-invasive and is being increasingly applied to the study of the heart. Spin echo images using cardiac gated acquisition have the advantage that moving blood has no signal giving excellent contrast compared to the surrounding soft tissues. Images can be acquired in orthogonal or oblique planes, and up to 16 can be produced within 3 to 4 minutes depending on heart rate. Useful information can be obtained in a variety of conditions including lesions of the myocardium, aorta and pericardium, the detection of tumours and thrombus and the complete display of anatomy in patients with congenital heart disease, both pre- and postoperatively. Although its place in the investigation of heart disease is still being established, already it can be regarded as an imaging technique complementary to echocardiography, which has partially replaced diagnostic invasive angiography and may eventually replace it completely.

Magnetic resonance is firmly established in imaging of the central nervous and musculoskeletal systems because of the quality of the images and the natural contrast between different tissues. The special advantages of magnetic resonance are not only the excellent spatial resolution in any orthogonal or oblique plane, and the wide range of contrast between different soft tissues, but also the variation of the parameters displayed in the images according to the biochemical environment. In recent years there has been increasing interest in cardiovascular magnetic resonance because despite the technical problems of imaging a moving organ, it is

0007–1420/89/0045–0933/$10.00

possible to obtain both anatomical and functional information and to avoid invasive investigation in some cases.[1–4] This chapter deals with anatomical display of cardiovascular disease using spin echo tomographic images, the advantage of which is that moving blood gives rise to no signal and provides good contrast between the vascular lumen and the surrounding soft tissues. On the other hand, motion of the heart presents a problem, and cardiac gating is essential to obtain high quality images. Acquisition of data is thus slow relative to the imaging of still organs, a typical image of 128x128 pixels with one repetition taking 256 cardiac cycles. However for anatomical display, multiple slices can be acquired simultaneously, so that up to 16 images can be produced within 3 to 4 minutes. Further functional information can be obtained with different sequences which provide cine imaging and flow measurements: these are described by Underwood in the next chapter.

MYOCARDIAL ANATOMY AND FUNCTION

Unlike radiographic images which are spatially distorted because of the non-parallel beam of radiation, magnetic resonance images have been shown to be dimensionally accurate.[5] It is therefore a simple exercise to measure the volume of a chamber by summing the areas in contiguous images. Ventricular stroke volumes can be measured from a set of transverse images at end systole and end diastole, and a set of eight pairs involve an acquisition time of about 30 minutes. Volume measurement by this method is independent of cavity shape unlike other methods where geometric assumptions usually have to be made. However because these are not too inaccurate for the left ventricle, a more rapid method of volume measurement for this chamber is by area-length calculations on oblique images containing the long axis of the ventricle.[6,7] For the irregularly shaped right ventricle, the multislice method is needed and it is then possible to calculate the regurgitant fraction in patients with valve regurgitation from left and right ventricular stroke volume differences.[8] This technique is only valid if a single valve is affected but it can be used in conjunction with cine imaging which gives a semiquantitative assessment of regurgitation through individual valves. Similarly, the pulmonary to systemic flow ratio can be calculated in patients with atrial or aortopulmonary shunts. Muscle volume and hence mass can also be measured on similar principles[9–15] and is particularly interesting in patients with left ventricular hypertrophy. For example it has been possible to show regression of hypertrophy following only three months treatment of hypertension.[16] Wall thickness in hypertrophic cardiomyopathy is better demonstrated than by echocardiography because the three dimensional distribution is more easily seen (Fig. 1).[17] Muscle thinning and aneurysm formation are also readily recognized (Fig. 2), and previous infarction can be detected and quantified by the presence and extent of thinning[18] and wall motion abnormality measured from diastolic and systolic images by superimposition of endocardial contours.[19,20]

THE AORTA

The aorta is particularly well seen because of its size, relative immobility and natural contrast between the wall and moving blood.[21-24] Aortic dissection is readily detected (Fig. 3) and its extent displayed including involvement of other vessels. The entry

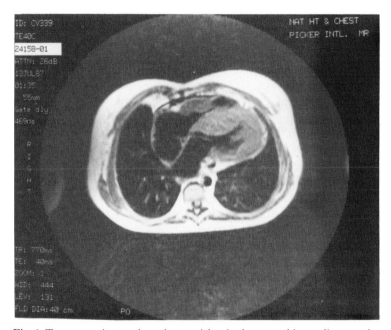

Fig. 1 Transverse image through ventricles in hypertrophic cardiomyopathy showing gross asymmetric hypertrophy involving the septum, left ventricular apex and anterior free wall of right ventricle.

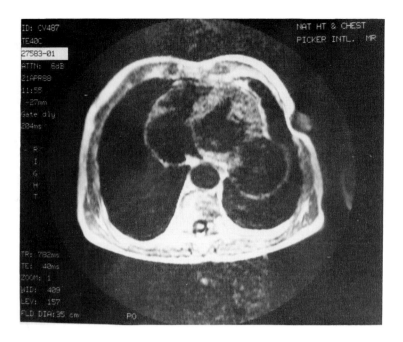

Fig. 2 Transverse image through left ventricle in patient following myocardial infarction. A large posterior aneurysm is present with a thin wall and narrow neck. At operation this was confirmed to be a false aneurysm of the left ventricle.

and exit points are more difficult to localize, but there is no doubt that invasive investigation can be avoided with a combination of echocardiography and magnetic resonance.[25] The previous inability to detect involvement of the aortic valve is no longer a problem, since aortic regurgitation can be detected and quantified on a cine sequence, and although an adequate assessment of the coronary arteries is not obtained, this is not always necessary preoperatively. The relative merits of magnetic resonance and computed tomography have been compared,[26] and it seems likely that the two investigations are equivalent in their sensitivity. Magnetic resonance had the advantage of oblique planes and does not require contrast injection, but it is more difficult to image sick patients in the current generation of scanners. The investigation performed in most cases will depend upon practical problems such as whether magnetic resonance is available. Other aortic abnormalities that are well seen by magnetic resonance are aneurysms,[27] stenoses including coarctation[28] and other congenital abnormali-

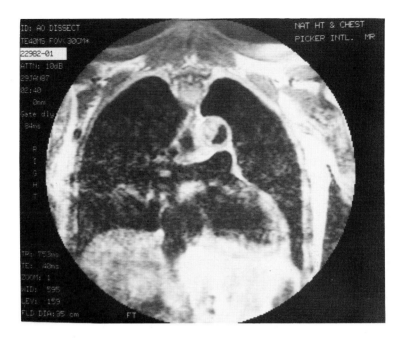

Fig. 3 Coronal image through aortic arch showing aortic dissection. The false lumen has a high signal from the slowly moving blood within it and there is no signal from the fast moving blood in the true lumen.

ties[29-31] and it is an ideal method for the long term follow-up of patients following coarctation repair and patients with Marfan's syndrome.[32,33] Spin echo images can also be used to assess the patency of coronary bypass grafts,[34-37] but although lack of signal in the lumen indicates some flowing blood, it may not bear any relationship to the effective flow which is better assessed by cine imaging and phase mapping. Another application of multislice imaging is in suspected abscess in the heart or around the aortic root in postoperative patients with infection which is difficult to control. Echocardiography is often equivocal in such patients and spin echo images will usually produce a definitive answer.[38]

THROMBUS AND TUMOURS

A common reason for referral for magnetic resonance imaging is to adjudicate upon the presence of intracardiac filling defects. Tumours of the heart and surrounding structures are well demonstrated (Fig. 4),[39-43] but with the possible exception of

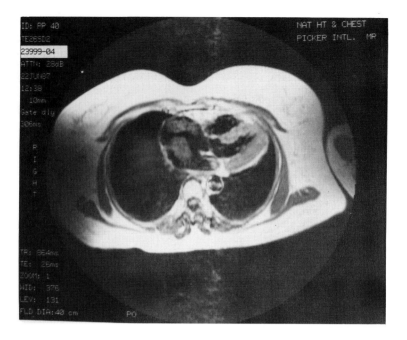

Fig. 4 Transverse image showing lobulated masses in the right atrium. At operation, these were found to be a haemangiopericytoma spreading from the primary in the kidney.

lipomata (high signal)[44] and fibromata (low signal), it can be difficult to distinguish different tumours. This is not a problem restricted to cardiology, since it has not been possible to characterize cerebral or hepatic lesions by their relaxation times, and although the morphological appearances usually give clues, it is disappointing that it can sometimes be difficult to tell a cystic lesion from a solid one. Thrombus is the commonest intracavitary filling defect and it is readily seen using a spin echo sequence. Confusion between thrombus and slowly moving blood can be avoided by using a cine sequence, where blood gives high signal and the thrombus appears as a filling defect.[45] On the topic of vascular imaging, there has been some interest in the detection of venous thrombus[46,47] and pulmonary emboli,[48] but it appears unlikely that magnetic resonance will prove to be sensitive in the detection of pulmonary emboli without both respiratory and cardiac gating.

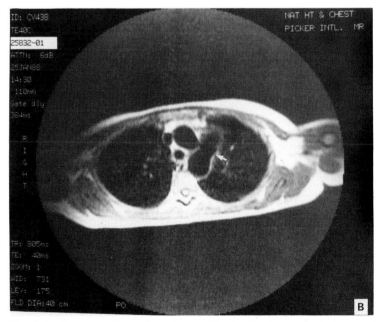

Fig. 5 A. Transverse image through ventricle showing large ventricular septal defect. **B.** Transverse image through aorta showing lumen of large ductus (arrow) connecting distal aortic arch to roof of pulmonary trunk.

THE PERICARDIUM

The normal fibrous pericardium appears as a thin dark line around the heart using a short spin echo sequence, and it is usually most easily seen anteriorly.[49] Pericardial thickening and effusion can be seen although the appearances of both depend upon the pathology. Thickened pericardium usually has a low signal, although it may have an intermediate or high signal, presumably if there is active inflammation with cellular infiltration and oedema.[50] In contrast to computed tomography, pericardial calcification is not demonstrated. Pericardial fluid usually has a high signal although it may lose signal with motion. The result is that it can be difficult to distinguish pericardium from fluid. The functional difference between constriction and restriction cannot be appreciated but in the former, abnormal pericardium is invariably seen, and in the latter it is not.[51]

CONGENITAL HEART DISEASE

This is another area where invasive investigation can be avoided in selected cases.[52,53] It is possible to detect lesions causing left-to-right shunts including ventricular and atrial septal defects and patent ductus (Fig. 5),[54] although specificity for the detection of atrial defects is a matter of debate.[55] Our own experience is that specificity using conventional imaging in the transverse plane is not very good, but in practice, the debate will be eclipsed by different techniques such as the use of oblique planes, cine imaging and velocity mapping. The strength of magnetic resonance in the assessment of septal defects is not so much in detecting the lesion (which will usually have been found by echocardiography), but in assessing its functional significance by measurements of flow through the shunt. Abnormalities of the atrioventricular valves are well seen,[56] but again, magnetic resonance is of greatest value in assessing functional sequelae such as ventricular contraction, regurgitation and flow. Magnetic resonance imaging is particularly suitable for the display of anatomy in cyanotic and

Fig. 6 Transverse images in double outlet right ventricle with pulmonary stenosis and bilateral Blalock shunts. **A.** Slice through the ventricles which are connected via a septal defect. **B.** Slice through the aortic root lying to the right of the narrow outflow to the pulmonary artery. **C.** Slice above showing hypoplastic pulmonary arteries (arrows). **D.** Slice through aortic arch showing small but patent Blalock shunts (arrows). The lack of signal in the lumen confirms their patency. (A = aorta, LV = left ventricle, RV = right ventricle, S = superior vena cava).

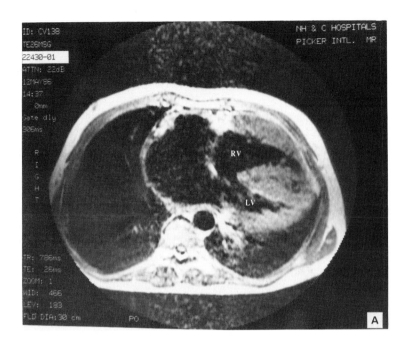

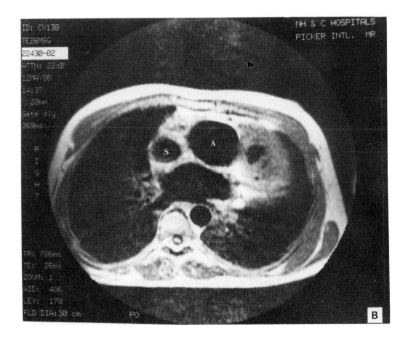

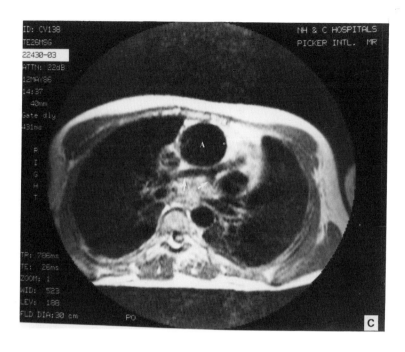

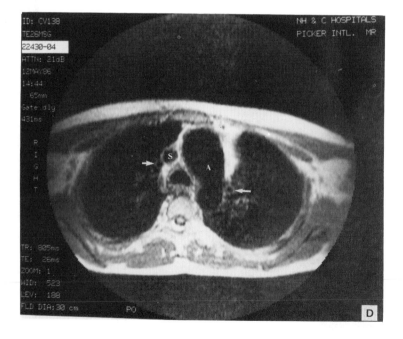

complex congenital heart disease. Venous, atrial, ventricular, outlet and arterial anatomy and connections can all be shown with the acquisition of multiple slices in the three orthogonal planes. The images have a striking clarity which is superior to two dimensional echocardiography and less dependent on operator skill and experience (Fig. 6). However in practical terms, the examinations are complimentary and magnetic resonance should not be regarded as a potential replacement for echocardiography but as a method of completing the anatomical assessment and rendering catheterisation and angiography unnecessary. In pulmonary atresia, the presence and state of the central pulmonary arteries and of systemic collaterals to the lungs is important, but this information can be very difficult to obtain, and magnetic resonance has reduced the number of invasive investigations in these patients.[57] Perhaps the most useful application of magnetic resonance in complex congenital heart disease is in the assessment of patients post-operatively. For example in transposition of the

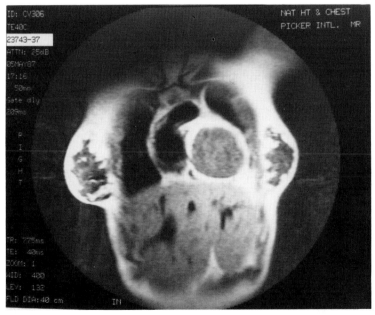

Fig. 7 Coronal image in patient following Fontan's operation for tricuspid atresia. There is intimal thickening narrowing the lumen of the conduit which was confirmed to be causing significant obstruction at reoperation.

great arteries following Mustard's operation, right ventricular and tricuspid valve function are important determinants of long term morbidity and these can be assessed repeatedly and non-invasively by magnetic resonance imaging.[58] Surgical conduits can also be clearly seen and accurate measurements of the lumen made and compared at subsequent studies to detect early evidence of obstruction (Fig.7). Magnetic resonance is therefore an important method of following up patients after Fontan's operation and its modifications and all patients with ventriculopulmonary conduits inserted for the correction of Fallot's tetralogy, pulmonary atresia, double outlet and truncus arteriosus. Magnetic resonance images have also been obtained in neonates and infants with congenital heart disease. A field strength of 1.5T offers the advantage of a higher signal to noise ratio and allows the acquisition of thin slices to provide the higher resolution needed to image small hearts. Sedation is also required but encouraging results have been reported which can lead to a reduction of invasive investigation in these patients.[59] In the future the development of rapid imaging techniques will be of considerable help in this area.[60]

REFERENCES

1 Steiner RE. Regular review; nuclear magnetic resonance imaging. Br Med J 1987; 294: 1570.
2 Pohost GM, Canby RC. Nuclear magnetic resonance imaging: current applications and future prospects. Circulation 1987; 75: 88–95.
3 Chambron J, Sacrez A, Mossard JM, Baruthio J, Germain P. La Résonance magnétique nucléaire. Notre expérience préliminaire sur le coeur normal et dans diverses cardiopathies. Ann Cardiol Angéiol 1986; 35: 67–73.
4 Casolo GC, Petacchi D, Bartolozzi C. L'‘imaging' cardiaco con la risonanza magnetica nucleare. G Ital Cardiol 1986, 16: 826–834.
5 Longmore DB, Klipstein RH, Underwood SR et al. Dimensional accuracy of magnetic resonance in studies of the heart. Lancet 1985; i: 1360–1362.
6 Osbakken M, Yuschok T. Evaluation of ventricular function with gated cardiac magnetic resonance imaging. Cathet Cardiovasc Diagn 1986, 12: 156–160.
7 Buckwalter KA, Aisen AM, Dilworth LR, Mancini GBJ, Buda AJ: Gated cardiac MRI: ejection fraction determination using the right anterior oblique view. Am J Roentgenol 1986; 147: 33–37.
8 Underwood SR, Klipstein RH, Firmin DN et al. Magnetic resonance assessment of aortic and mitral regurgitation. Br Heart J 1986; 56: 455–462.
9 Florentine MS, Grosskreutz CL, Chang W et al. Measurement of left ventricular mass in vivo using gated nuclear magnetic resonance imaging. J Am Coll Cardiol 1986; 8: 107–112.
10 Keller AM, Peshock RM, Malloy CR, Buja LM, Nunnally R, Parkey RW, Willerson JT. In vivo measurement of myocardial mass using nuclear magnetic resonance imaging. J Am Coll Cardiol, 1986; 8: 113–117.
11 Caputo GR, Tscholakoff D, Sechtem U, Higgins CB. Measurement of canine left ventricular mass by using MR imaging. Am J Roentgenol 1987; 148: 33–38.

12 Katz J, Milliken MC, Stray-Gundersen J et al. Estimation of human myocardial mass with MR imaging. Radiology 1988; 169: 495–498.

13 Milliken MC, Stray-Gundersen J, Peshock RM, Katz J, Mitchell JH. Left ventricular mass as determined by magnetic resonance imaging in male endurance athletes. Am J Cardiol 1988; 62: 301–305.

14 Just H, Holubarsch C, Friedburg H. Estimation of left ventricular volume and mass by magnetic resonance imaging: comparison with quantitative biplane angiography. Cardiovasc Intervent Radiol 1987; 10: 1–4.

15 Maddahi J, Crues J, Berman DS et al. Noninvasive quantification of left ventricular myocardial mass by gated proton nuclear magnetic resonance imaging. J Am Coll Cardiol 1987; 10:682–692.

16 Eichstädt HW, Felix R, Langer M et al. Use of nuclear magnetic resonance imaging to show regression of hypertrophy with ramipril treatment. Am J Cardiol 1987; 59: 98D–103D.

17 Berghöfer G, Köhler D, Schmutzler H, Schneider R, Felix R. Die magnetresonanz-tomographische Darstellung bei hypertropher Kardiomyopathie im Vergleich zur Echokardiographie. Herz/Kreisl 1987; 19: 135–139.

18 Akins AW, Hill JA, Sievers KW, Conti CR. Assessment of left ventricular wall thickness in healed myocardial infarction by magnetic resonance imaging. Am J Cardiol 1987; 59: 24–28.

19 Underwood SR, Rees RSO, Savage PE et al. The assessment of regional left ventricular function by magnetic resonance. Br Heart J 1986; 56: 334–340.

20 Akins EW, Hill JA, Sievers KW, Conti CR: Assessment of left ventricular wall thickness is healed myocardial infarction by magnetic resonance imaging. Am J Cardiol 1987; 59: 24–28.

21 Dooms GC, Higgins CB. The potential of magnetic resonance imaging for the evaluation of thoracic arterial disease. J Thorac Cardiovasc Surg 1986; 92: 1088–1095.

22 Mossard JM, Baruthio J, Germain P. Apport de la résonance magnétique nucléaire dans le diagnostic des affections aortiques. Arch Mal Coeur 1986; 79: 456–461.

23 Kersting-Sommerhoff BA, Higgins CS, White RD, Sommerhoff CP, Lipton MJ. Aortic dissection: Sensitivity and specificity of MR imaging. Radiology 1988; 166: 651–655.

24 Pernes JM, Grenier P, Desbleds MT, de Brux JL. MR evaluation of chronic aortic dissection. J Comput Assist Tomogr 1987; 11: 975–981.

25 Goldman AP, Kotler MN, Scanlon MH, Ostrum BJ, Parameswaran R, Parry WR. Magnetic resonance imaging and two dimensional echocardiography. Alternative approach to aortography in diagnosis of aortic dissection aneurysm. Am J Med 1986; 80: 1225–1229.

26 Goldman AP, Kotler MN, Scanlon MH, Ostrum B, Parameswaran R, Parry WR. The complementary role of magnetic resonance imaging, Doppler echocardiography, and computed tomography in the diagnosis of dissecting thoracic aneurysms. Am Heart J 1986, 111: 970–981.

27 Winkler M, Higgins CB. MRI of perivalvular infectious pseudoaneurysms. Am J Roentgenol 1986, 147: 253–256.

28 Boxer RA, Fishman MC, LaCorte MA, Singh S, Parnell VA Jr. Diagnosis and postoperative evaluation of supravalvular aortic stenosis by magnetic resonance imaging. Am J Cardiol 1986; 58: 367–368.

29 Biset GS, Strife JL, Kirks DR, Bailey WW. Vascular rings: MR imaging. Am J Roentgenol 1987; 149: 251–256.

30 Brown K, Batra P. MR imaging of aneurysm of an aberrant right subclavian artery. J Comput Assist Tomogr 1987; 11: 1071–1073.

31 Gomes AS, Lois JF, George B, Alpan G, Williams RG. Congenital abnormalities of the aortic arch: MR imaging. Radiology 1987; 165: 691–695.

32 Schaefer S, Peshock RM, Mallot CR, Katz J, Parkey RW, Willerson JT:

Nuclear magnetic resonance imaging in Marfan's syndrome. J Am Coll Cardiol 1987, 9: 70–74.

33 Boxer RA, LaCorte MA, Singh S, Davis J, Goldman M, Stein HL: Evaluation of the aorta in the Marfan syndrome by magnetic resonance imaging. Am Heart J 1986, 111: 1001–1002.

34 Jenkins JPR, Love HG, Foster CJ, Isherwood I, Rowlands DJ. Detection of coronary artery bypass graft patency as assessed by magnetic resonance imaging. Br J Radiol 1988; 61: 2–4.

35 Gomes AS, Lois JF, Drinkwater DC Jr, Corday SR. Coronary artery bypass grafts: visualization with MR imaging. Radiology 1987; 162: 175–9.

36 Rubinstein RI, Askenase AD, Thickman D, Feldman MS, Agarwal JB, Helfant RH. Magnetic resonance imaging to evaluate patency of aortocoronary bypass grafts. Circulation 1987; 76: 786–791.

37 White RD, Caputo GR, Mark AS, Modin GW, Higgins CB. Coronary artery bypass graft patency: noninvasive evaluation with MR imaging. Radiology 1987; 164: 681–686.

38 Miller SW, Palmer EL, Dinsmore RE, Brady TJ. Gallium-67 and magnetic resonance imaging in aortic root abscess J Nucl Med 1987; 28: 1616–1619.

39 Applegate PM, Tajik AJ, Ehman RL, Julsrud PR, Miller FA Jr. Two-dimensional echocardiographic and magnetic resonance imaging observations in massive lipomatous hypertrophy of the atrial septum. Am J Cardiol 1987; 59: 489–491.

40 Conti VR, Saydjari R, Amparo EG. Paraganglioma of the heart. The value of magnetic resonance imaging in the preoperative evaluation. Chest 1986; 90: 604–606.

41 Grötz J, Steiner G, Josephs W, Sorge B, Wiechmann W, Beyer HK. Darstellung intra- und parakardialer raumfordernder Prozesse mit der magnetischen Resonanztomographie. Dtsch med Wochenschr 1986; 111: 1594–1598.

42 Freedberg RS, Kronzon I, Rumancik WM, Leibeskind D. The contribution of magnetic resonance imaging to the evaluation of intracardiac tumours diagnosed by echocardiography. Circulation 1988; 77: 96–103.

43 Winkler M, Higgins CB. Suspected intracardiac masses: evalution with MR imaging. Radiology 1987; 165: 117–122.

44 Applegate PM, Tajik AJ, Ehman RL, Julsrud PR, Miller FA Jr. Two-dimensional echocardiographic and magnetic resonance imaging observations in massive lipomatous hypertophy of the atrial septum. Am J Cardiol 1987; 59: 489–91.

45 Dinsmore RE, Wedeen V, Rosen B, Wismer GL, Miller SW, Brandy TJ. Phase-offset technique to distinguish slow blood flow and thrombus on MR images. Am J Roentgenol 1987; 148: 634–636.

46 Erdman WA, Weinreb JC, Cohen JM, Buja LM, Chaney C, Peshock RM. Venous thrombosis: clinical and experimental MR imaging. Radiology 1986, 161: 233–238.

47 Rapoport S, Sostman HD, Pope C, Camputaro CM, Holcomb W, Gore JC. Venous clots: Evaluation with MR imaging. Radiology 1987; 162: 527–530.

48 Stein MG, Crues JV III, Bradley WG Jr et al. MR imaging of pulmonary emboli: an experimental study in dogs. Am J Roentgenol 1986, 147: 1133–1137.

49 Sechtem U, Tscholakoff D, Higgins CB. MRI of the normal pericardium. Am J Roentgenol 1986; 147: 239–244.

50 Sechtem U, Tscholakoff D, Higgins CB. MRI of the abnormal pericardium. Am J Roentgenol 1986; 147: 245–252.

51 Sechtem U, Higgins CB, Sommerhoff BA, Lipton MJ, Huycke EC. Magnetic resonance imaging of restrictive cardiomyopathy. Am J Cardiol 1987, 59: 480–482.

52 Boxer RA, Singh S, LaCorte MA, Goldman M, Stein HL. Cardiac magnetic

resonance imaging in children with congenital heart disease. J Paediatr 1986; 109: 460–464.

53 Wolff F, Baruthio J, Wecker D, Brechenmacher C, Chambron J: Apport de l'imagerie par résonance magnétique dans les cardiopathies congénitales. Arch Mal Coeur 1986; 79: 1563–1568.

54 Didier D, Higgins CB: Identification and localisation of ventricular septal defect by gated magnetic resonance imaging. Am J Cardiol 1986; 57: 1363–1368.

55 Diethelm L, Déry R, Lipton MJ, Higgins CB: Atrial-level shunts: sensitivity and specificity of MR in diagnosis. Radiology 1987; 162: 181–186.

56 Fletcher BD, Jacobstein MD, Abramowsky CR, Anderson RH: Right atrioventricular valve atresia: anatomic evaluation with MR imaging. Am J Radiol 1987; 148: 671–674.

57 Rees RSO, Somerville J, Underwood SR, Wright J, Firmin DN, Klipstein RH, Longmore DB. Magnetic resonance imaging of the pulmonary arteries and their systemic connections in pulmonary atresia: comparison with angiographic and surgical findings. Br Heart J 1987; 58: 621–6.

58 Rees RSO, Jane Somerville, Carol Warnes, SR Underwood, DN Firmin, RH Klipstein, DB Longmore. Comparison of magnetic resonance imaging with echocardiography and radionuclide angiography in assessing cardiac function and anatomy following Mustard's operation for transposition of the great arteries. Am J Cardiol 1988; 61: 1316–22.

59 Smith MA, Baker EJ, Ayton VT, Parsons JM, Ladusans EJ, Maisey MN. Magnetic resonance imaging of the infant heart at 1.5T. Br J Radiol 1989; 62: 367–70.

60 Rzedzian RR, Pykett IL. Instant images of the human heart using a new, whole-body MR imaging system. Am J Roentgenol 1987; 149: 245–250.

British Medical Bulletin (1989) Vol. 45, No. 4, pp. 948–967
© The British Council 1989

Cine magnetic resonance imaging and flow measurements in the cardiovascular system

S R Underwood
National Heart & Lung Institute, London

CINE IMAGING

Conventional magnetic resonance imaging using spin echo sequences produces static images at chosen points of the cardiac cycle. These images demonstrate cardiac anatomy well but some aspects of function are best evaluated by cine imaging. Cine imaging is available on most commercial scanners and it is being increasingly used for the assessment of cardiac function, valvular function, and for the measurement of blood flow.

Technical considerations

As already described in this issue (Longmore), magnetic resonance images are constructed from a number of data acquisitions, each with a different phase encoding gradient. A typical number of acquisitions for cardiac imaging is 128 and these may be acquired twice and averaged. Each acquisition contributes to a line of the image, although the line is in frequency or 'K' space and not in real space. For cardiac imaging, only one acquisition can be triggered per cycle since all the acquisitions must correspond to the same part of the cycle. Total imaging time is therefore 256 cycles or three to four minutes depending upon heart rate.

For cine acquisition, the selected plane is excited many times per cycle but each excitation contributes to a different image. At the end of 256 cycles a number of images is produced corresponding to different parts of the cycle. The repetition time of the sequence must equal the required temporal resolution and is

0007–1420/89/0045–0948/$10.00

typically between 10 ms and 50 ms. If the usual 90° excitation pulse is used, the imaging plane would become magnetically saturated and little or no signal would be obtained, but by reducing the excitation flip angle to between 20° and 45° this problem can be overcome. Using this technique, cine spin echo images have been acquired with a temporal resolution of 12 frames per cardiac cycle.[1]

The spin echo sequence is not ideal for such rapid repetition and much greater success has been achieved using variants of the field echo (or gradient refocussed echo) sequence, which have become known by acronyms such as FEER, GRASS, FAST, and FLASH. In these sequences, magnetic field gradients are used to dephase and then rephase the protons following an excitation pulse, and an echo is produced much more rapidly than by using a 180° pulse. Reduced flip angles are used for the initial exciting pulse to avoid saturation. An additional manoeuvre to maintain signal from moving blood is to make use of the 'even echo rephasing' phenomenon and to acquire the second echo rather than the first. Echo times of 6 ms and repeat times of 10 ms can be attained in commercial magnetic resonance scanners and in experimental small bore machines echo times of 1 ms and repeat times of 3 ms have been achieved.

For clinical imaging, 32 frames per cardiac cycle is adequate but 16 frames are often used so that the repeat time is not greater than 30 or 50 ms. Excitation need not be in a single plane and, for instance, with 48 excitations per cardiac cycle 4 different planes can be imaged with 12 frames per cycle in each.

One of the main features of spin echo images is the high contrast between soft tissues. With the very rapid repetition times of cine field echo sequences this contrast is lost because adequate time for longitudinal relaxation (and hence T1 contrast) is not available. Contrast between blood and myocardium is maintained, however, because fresh unmagnetized blood is continuously flowing through the plane. If flow is inadequate then contrast is lost and this occurs particularly in the vertical and horizontal long axis planes where flow is mainly in the plane of the image. Contrast in the short axis plane is usually good.

Ventricular function

Cine display of the left ventricle allows systolic function to be evaluated subjectively from wall motion and wall thickening.

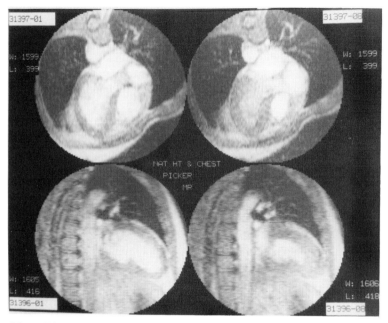

Fig. 1 Diastolic (left) and systolic (right) cine FEER images in horizontal long axis (top) and vertical long axis planes (bottom) in a normal subject.

Figure 1 shows diastolic and systolic images through the left ventricle in a normal subject. Wall thickening is uniform and motion is concentric. In patients with coronary artery disease, wall motion is often normal in the absence of previous infarction, but abnormalities may be induced by intravenous dipyridamole which is a powerful coronary arterial dilator increasingly used as an adjunct to dynamic exercise in thallium-201 myocardial perfusion imaging. Although the mechanism is complex, it may induce ischaemia and wall motion abnormalities in a proportion of patients with coronary artery disease. Figure 2 shows an example.

Although the cine display is frequently assessed subjectively, more reliable measurements can be made of ventricular volumes and of muscle thickness and thickening between end diastole and end systole. Ventricular volumes are most accurately measured by summing areas in multiple contiguous sections, and several studies have successfully compared the results with angiography[2] and echocardiography.[3] In theory, it does not matter which plane is used for the measurements, but the short axis plane appears to be the best because of the good contrast between blood and myocar-

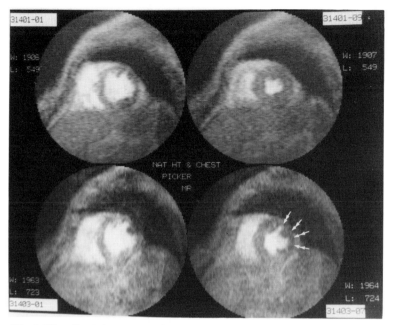

Fig. 2 Diastolic (left) and systolic (right) short axis images in a patient with coronary artery disease without previous infarction, before (above) and following (below) intravenous dipyridamole. Hypokinesis and failure to thicken are induced in the anterolateral wall (arrows).

dium. The technique is time consuming, however, since definition of the blood pool in each image has to be performed manually. Much more rapid measurements can be made using the area-length technique in either a single plane or in two perpendicular planes. The area-length technique assumes that the ventricle is an ellipsoid of revolution about its long axis and although this is a reasonable assumption in normal ventricles, significant errors can be made in ventricles with regional abnormalities.[4]

The main difficulty when studying regional left ventricular wall motion is the distinction between active contraction and passive motion caused by translation and rotation. Many different methods have been used and whilst none is ideal, the centre-line technique is probably the best. This uses a fixed external reference system and measures motion along a line perpendicular to the centre-line between the diastolic and the systolic endocardial contours. Because of these problems, wall thickening between diastole and systole is preferable to wall motion alone when considering regional function.[5] The short axis plane is ideal and the effect of previous infarction is readily detected and quantified.[6]

More sophisticated measures of left ventricular function can also be derived by calculating wall stress. End systolic stress can be calculated as: $(1.35 \times P \times D)/4 \times (1 + h/D)$, where P is the end systolic left ventricular pressure in millimetres of mercury which is assumed from measuring the blood pressure, D is the end systolic diameter of the ventricle in centimetres, and h is the end systolic wall thickness in centimetres. Such measurements in patients with a varity of conditions have provided interesting results, which may be valuable for assessing therapeutic responses. Patients with secondary left ventricular hypertrophy have wall stress comparable with that of normal subjects, but patients with valvular regurgitation have high stress in proportion to the severity of regurgitation. In dilated cardiomyopathy, wall stress is also increased but ejection fraction is much less than those in patients with regurgitation and comparable wall stress.[7]

Valvular function

Cine magnetic resonance imaging provides a number of methods for assessing valvular function. If left and right ventricular volumes are measured at end diastole and end systole, any discrepancy between the stroke volumes must be due to regurgitation and the regurgitant fraction can be calculated as (LVSV–RVSV)/LVSV.[8] This is a particularly accurate technique as has been shown by a comparison of stroke volumes in normal subjects where left and right ventricular stroke volumes should be almost identical.[9] If more than one valve is regurgitant then the regurgitant fraction is the mean of that from both valves, unless they are on opposite sides when accurate quantification is impossible. The comparison between regurgitant fraction and other methods of measuring regurgitation has already been covered (Rees, this issue) but the technique appears to be equally accurate whether spin echo images[8] or cine field echo images[10] are used.

A second method by which valvular regurgitation can be assessed is measurement of the area of signal loss produced by the turbulent jet. As discussed by Longmore (this issue), the FEER sequence and related sequences give high signal from blood unless it is turbulent, when signal is lost. The presence of acceleration and higher orders of motion in a pixel produces the signal loss, and these higher orders are present in the turbulent vortices of regurgitant jets or distal to a stenosis or other vascular abnormality. Although this signal loss may not correspond exactly with turbulence, its size has been used to provide a semi-quantitative estimate of regurgitation through individual valves.[11,12] The extent of turbulence can either be expressed as an absolute volume or more conveniently by grading the size of the jet. We have shown that a simple grading system agrees approximately with the conventional grading system used in angiocardiography, with grade 1 being signal loss close to the valve, grade 2 extending into the proximal chamber, grade 3 filling the whole of the proximal chamber, and grade 4 if the receiving chamber has signal loss throughout the whole of the relevant half of the cardiac cycle.[11] Figure 3 shows a patient with grade 2 rheumatic mitral regurgitation.

It was hoped that the same method of quantifying regurgitation could be used to measure valvular stenosis, but results have been unreliable. Although in phantom experiments the size of the turbulent area downstream from a stenosis is related to the

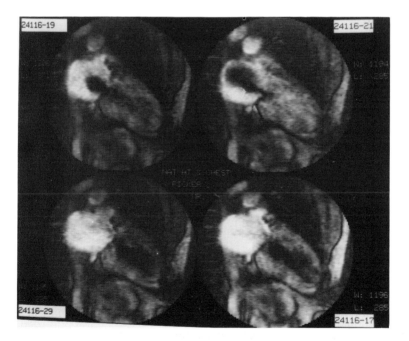

Fig. 3 Four frames from a cine acquisition in the vertical long axis plane in a patient with rheumatic mitral stenosis and regurgitation. The turbulent jet is clearly seen as a signal void in the left atrium during systole, and there is also diastolic turbulence in the left ventricle in diastole because of the stenosis.

gradient across it, in clinical applications other factors may lead to turbulence. A bicuspid but unstenosed aortic valve, for instance, may produce marked turbulence. The area of signal loss also depends upon the sequence used and sequences with shorter echo times are much less susceptible to turbulence. This is illustrated in Figure 4 where there is marked systolic signal loss distal to a bicuspid aortic valve using the FEER sequence with an echo time of 14 ms, but no signal loss using 6 ms. Whether sequences with very short echo times will allow stenoses to be measured is still to be tested although preliminary results in the right heart are encouraging (see Fig. 5).

FLOW IMAGING

Technical considerations

The available techniques for measuring flow by magnetic resonance have been reviewed by Longmore earlier in this issue.

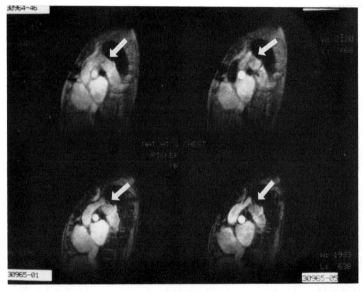

Fig. 4 This patient has aortic coarctation (arrowed) and a bicuspid but unstenosed aortic valve. On the left are diastolic frames and on the right systole. The upper images had echo time of 14 ms and the lower images 6 ms. There is systolic signal loss using the longer echo time in the ascending aorta and also distal to the coarctation at the entry of a collateral vessel. With the 6 ms sequence signal is preserved throughout the aorta. No turbulence is seen distal to the coarctation because it was very tight with little flow across it.

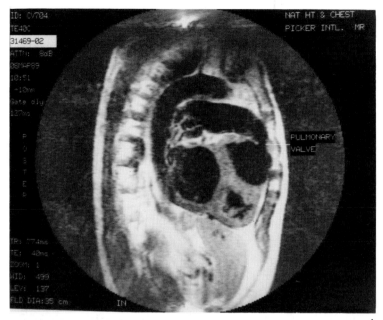

A

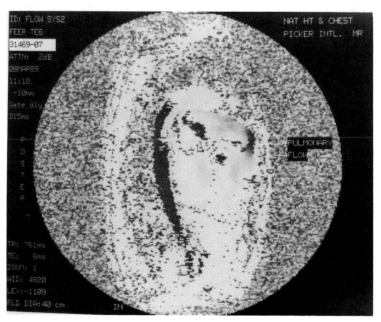

B

Although a number of techniques is available, encoding of the phase of the magnetic resonance signal with velocity at each point in the imaging plane is the only one to have achieved clinical application to date. There are a number of relevant technical considerations.

If no signal is obtained from blood then it is impossible to measure velocity since phase is meaningless in the absence of amplitude. This produces problems in a number of situations since although signal is nearly always obtained from normally flowing blood, abnormal flow patterns are frequently turbulent and lead to signal loss. It is difficult, for instance, to measure velocity in the orifice of a stenosed aortic valve and therefore difficult to compute the gradient across the valve. The ability to acquire images with very short echo times may overcome this problem but clinical experience is still limited. Figure 5 shows a patient with pulmonary stenosis in whom there was marked signal loss using the FEER sequence with an echo time of 14 ms. With an echo time of 6 ms however there was sufficient signal to produce a velocity map and to compute a gradient across the valve. It seems likely that gradients in excess of 50 mmHg will not be measured at 6 ms but with even shorter echo times higher gradients may be achieved.

Before acquiring a velocity map it is necessary to specify the range of velocities to be measured, thus the phase range of 0° to 360° might be used to encode velocities from 0 to 2 m/s. If velocities outside this range are encountered then the phenomenon of aliasing occurs and velocities above 2 m/s would appear the same as velocities above 0 m/s. Although the position of the velocity window can be altered after the acquisition to display velocities from 1 m/s to 3 m/s or from −1 m/s to +1 m/s, it is better to use an appropriate velocity window before the acquisition.

Cine velocity mapping allows flow in blood vessels such as the aorta and pulmonary to be measured with accuracy. Validation of the measurements has been made by comparison with Doppler

---

Fig. 5 This patient has pulmonary atresia and a homograft conduit to reconstruct the right ventricular outflow tract. The homograft valve had calcified and become stenotic and incompetent. (**a**) Sagittal spin echo image showing the pulmonary stenosis. (**b**) Systolic velocity map of the same slice encoded from bottom to top (inferior to superior). Rapid flow through the pulmonary valve is seen with a peak velocity of 3.2 m/s suggesting a gradient of 40 mmHg across the valve.

ultrasound,[13] but more importantly by an internal comparison of flow in the aorta, pulmonary artery, and left and right ventricular stroke volumes in normal subjects.[14,15] These four measurements should be the same apart from small differences due to coronary and bronchial flow and it can be calculated that flow measurements in large vessels are accurate to within approximately 6%. Accuracy is reduced in smaller vessels but it is still possible to make clinically useful measurements in arteries such as the femoral and carotid. Another factor which affects the accuracy of the measurements is the plane in which they are made. For greatest accuracy the vessel should be running perpendicularly through the plane of imaging and velocity should be encoded thorugh the plane. If the vessel is running in the plane of the image, it is still possible to encode velocities within it, but these may be lower than the true values because of partial volume effect and the inclusion of both stationary and static material in individual pixels.

Clinical applications

The most successful clinical application of velocity mapping has been in patients with congenital heart disease.[16] Intracardiac shunting can be measured in a number of ways. In an atrial septal defect the shunting can be assessed from the right and left ventricular stroke volumes but this method is not applicable in complex lesions or in ventricular shunts. Flow directly through ventricular defects can be visualised (Fig. 6), but the best method has been to measure aortic and pulmonary flow directly. This is also very helpful in complex lesions. Figure 7 shows a patient with truncus arteriosus. The possibility of surgery in such patients depends partly upon pulmonary flow which is difficult to measure by other techniques. Velocity mapping showed the ratio of pulmonary to systemic flow to be 0.65 and the patient was not submitted to surgery. Another complex congenital case is illustrated in Figure 8. The patient had an Eisenmenger patent ductus arteriosus with a small ventricular septal defect. From measurements of flow in the aorta, pulmonary artery and right and left

Fig. 6 (a) Spin echo image showing a large atrial septal defect. **(b)** Velocity map of the same slice encoded from bottom to top of the image (posterior to anterior). The flow through the defect is seen as well as flow within the aorta and pulmonary artery.

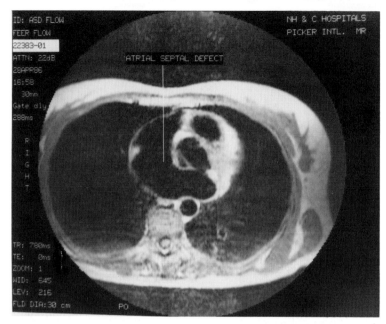

A

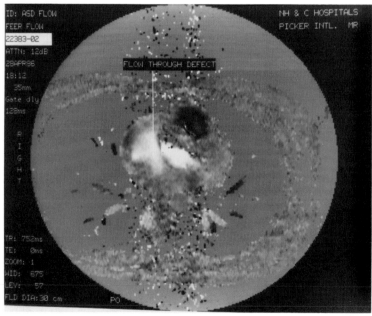

B

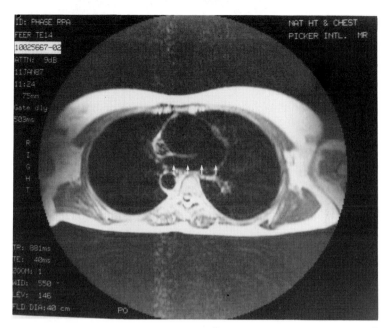

A

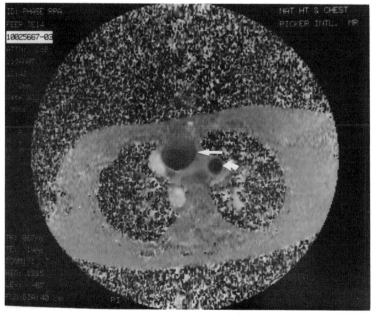

B

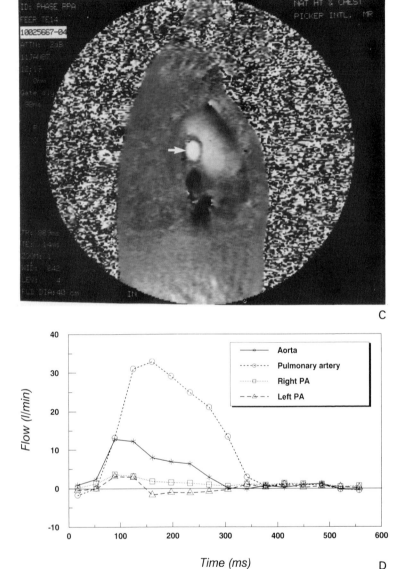

Fig. 7 (**a**) Transverse spin echo image in a patient with truncus arteriosus, showing the main and right pulmonary arteries arising posteriorly from the common arterial trunk (arrows). (**b**) Velocity map in a transverse plane slightly cranial to that of (a) showing flow in the aorta (arrow) and the left pulmonary artery (curved arrow). (**c**) Sagittal velocity map showing flow in the right pulmonary artery (arrow). (**d**) Flow profiles in each of the vessels demonstrating the low pulmonary to systemic flow ratio.

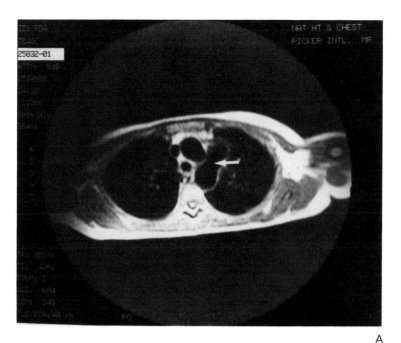

A

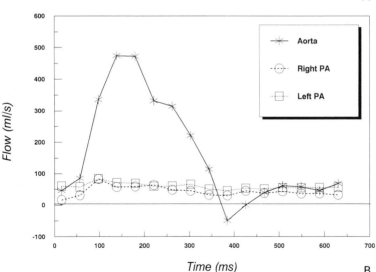

B

Fig. 8 (**a**) Transverse spin echo image showing a large patent ductus arteriosus (arrow) connecting the descending aorta to the pulmonary artery. The patient also had a ventricular septal defect and severe pulmonary hypertension. (**b**) Flow profiles in the major arteries from which shunting through each of the lesions could be calculated.

pulmonary arteries it was possible to calculate flow through each of the defects separately. Other structures of interest for the measurement of flow are surgically created shunts and conduits. Figure 9 shows a patient with transposition of the great arteries, pulmonary stenosis and a ventricular septal defect who had bilateral Blalock shunts created previously. Clinically, it was felt that the left sided shunt was patent since a murmur could be heard and Doppler echocardiography demonstrated flow within it, but the right sided shunt was thought to be occluded because neither a murmur nor Doppler flow could be demonstrated. Magnetic resonance imaging, however, clearly showed the patent right Blalock shunt and flow within it could be measured by velocity mapping.

Coronary artery bypass grafts are another potential application of magnetic resonance flow measurements. Conventional imaging

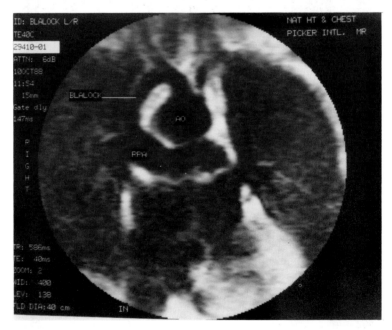

Fig. 9 Coronal spin echo imaging showing a right sided Blalock shunt connecting the right subclavian artery to the tight pulmonary artery in a patient with transposition of the great arteries, pulmonary stenosis and a ventricular septal defect. The shunt was thought to be occluded because there was no right murmur and Doppler echocardiography was unable to demonstrate flow within it. The magnetic resonance image shows it to be widely patent and velocity mapping was able to measure the flow within it.

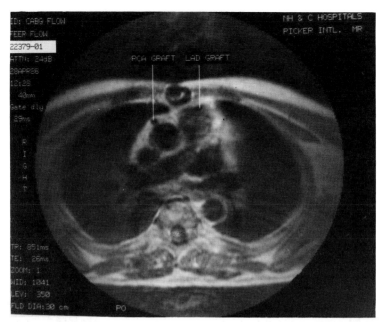

A

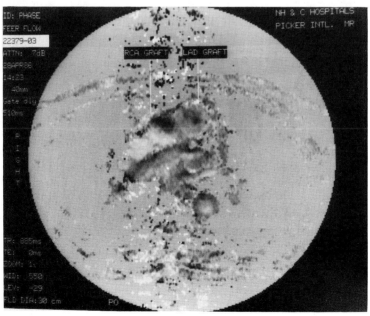

B

is able to identify patent grafts[17-21] but if it is possible to measure flow within the grafts this is much more valuable. Figure 10 shows a patient with grafts to the left anterior descending and right coronary arteries. The latter graft was known to be to a vessel that had undergone endarterectomy and had distal disease. Velocity mapping was able to demonstrate good flow within the left anterior descending graft but almost no flow in the right coronary graft. It is not possible to measure flow in all grafts however, and problems arise with artefact from sternal suture wires and from clips left during surgery. Metallic objects cause much larger artefacts in field echo sequences than in spin echo sequences and imaging of the grafts may be prevented altogether.

Coronary artery flow measurements can not yet be made reliably although good results can be obtained in favourable circumstances. Figure 11 shows coronary flow measurements in a patient with an anomalous left coronary artery arising from the pulmonary trunk. This had led to shunting from the aorta to the pulmonary artery through the right artery and around the apex into the low pressure system. The coronary flow profile showed a normal diastolic peak, presumably blood destined to nourish the myocardium, and an abnormal systolic peak which was thought to reflect the shunting. Flow measurements in coronary arteries of normal size are more difficult. The main problems are the tortuosity of the vessels and the gated nature of image acquisition. The former problem may be overcome by three dimensional acquisition and display techniques, and the latter by echo planar imaging in which an image is acquired almost in real time (30 ms acquisition). Echo planar imaging has been available on experimental magnetic resonance imagers for some time,[22,23] but it is only just becoming available on commercial machines.[24,25,26]

CONCLUSION

Cine magnetic resonance imaging provides additional functional information when compared with static spin echo images. Velocity mapping combined with cine imaging allow a comprehensive examination of the cardiovascular system, in some cases avoiding

---

Fig. 10 (a) Transverse spin echo image showing coronary bypass grafts to the left anterior descending and right coronary arteries. (**b**) The corresponding velocity map shows good flow in the left sided graft but no flow in the right sided graft.

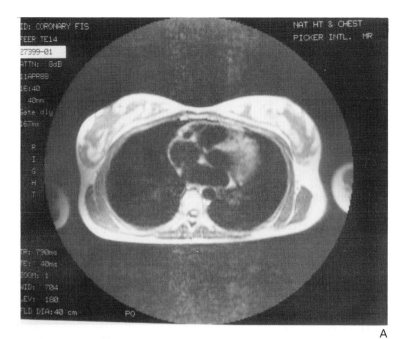

A

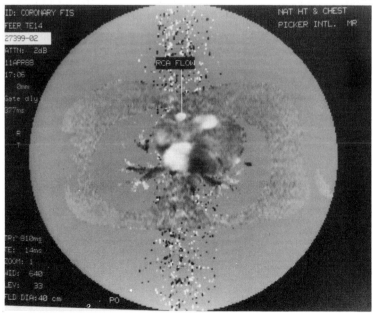

B

Fig. 11 (**a**) Spin echo image showing a dilated right coronary artery in a patient with anomalous left coronary artery arising from the pulmonary artery. (**b**) Velocity map showing coronary flow measurements.

the need for invasive catheterisation. The wider use of the techniques depends upon their availability but, as magnetic resonance imagers become more common, their use is likely to increase.

REFERENCES

1 Waterton JC, Jenkins JPR, Zhu XP, Love HG, Isherwood I, Rowlands DJ. Magnetic resonance (MR) cine imaging of the human heart. Br J Radiol 1985; 58: 711–716

2 Utz JA, Herfkens RJ, et al. Cine MRI determination of left ventricular ejection fraction. Am J Roentgenol 1987; 148: 839–843

3 Sechtem U, Pflugfelder PW, Gould RG, Cassidy MM, Higgins CB. Measurement of right and left ventricular volumes in healthy individuals with cine MR imaging. Radiology 1987; 163: 697–702

4 Underwood SR, Gill CRW, Firmin DN, et al. Left ventricular volume measured rapidly by oblique magnetic resonance imaging. Br Heart J 1988; 60: 188–195

5 Underwood SR, Rees RSO, Savage PE, et al. The assessment of regional left ventricular function by magnetic resonance. Br Heart J 1986; 56: 334–340

6 Pflugfelder PW, Sechtem UP, White RD, et al. Cine MRI: Quantitation of regional myocardial function by rapid cine MR imaging. Am J Roentgenol 1988; 150: 523–529

7 Holt WW, Wolfe C, Pflugfelder P, et al. Quantitation of left ventricular function by cine MR: Wall stress measurement in normal and cardiomyopathic subjects (Abstract). Society of Magnetic Resonance in Medicine, San Francisco, 1988; p. 136

8 Underwood SR, Klipstein RH, Firmin DN, et al. Magnetic resonance assessment of aortic and mitral regurgitation. Br Heart J 1986; 56: 455–462

9 Longmore DB, Klipstein RH, Underwood SR, et al. Dimensional accuracy of magnetic resonance in studies of the heart. Lancet 1985; i: 1360–1362

10 Sechtem U, Pflugfelder PW, Cassidy MM, et al. Mitral or aortic regurgitation: Quantification of regurgitant volumes with cine MR imaging. Radiology 1988; 167: 425–430

11 Underwood SR, Firmin DN, Mohiaddin RH, et al. Cine magnetic resonance imaging of valvular heart disease (Abstract). Society of Magnetic Resonance Imaging, New York, 1987; p. 723

12 Wagner S, Auffermann W, Buser P, et al. The signal void in cine MR accurately detects and grades severity of valvular regurgitation (Abstract). Society of Magnetic Resonance in Medicine, San Francisco, 1988; p. 201

13 Nayler GL, Firmin DN, Longmore DB. Blood Flow Imaging by Cine Magnetic Resonance. J Comput Assist Tomogr 1986; 10: 715–722

14 Firmin DN, Nayler GL, Klipstein RH, Underwood SR, Rees RSO, Longmore DB. In vivo validation of magnetic resonance velocity imaging. J Comput Assist Tomogr 1987; 11: 751–756

15 Bogren HG, Klipstein RH, Firmin DN, et al. Ante and retrograde blood flow distribution in the human ascending aorta analyzed by magnetic resonance. Am Heart J 1989 (In press)

16 Underwood SR, Firmin DN, Klipstein RH, Rees RSO, Longmore DB. Magnetic resonance velocity mapping: clinical application of a new technique. Br heart J 1987; 57: 404–412

17 Gomes AS, Lois JF, Drinkwater DC Jr, Corday SR. Coronary artery bypass grafts: visualization with MR imaging. Radiology 1987; 162: 175–179

18 Rubinstein RI, Askenase AD, Thickman D, Feldman MS, Agarwal JB, Helfant

RH. Magnetic resonance imaging to evaluate patency of aortocoronary bypass grafts. Circulation 1987; 76: 786–791

19 White RD, Caputo GR, Mark AS, Modin GW, Higgins CB. Coronary artery bypass graft patency: noninvasive evaluation with MR imaging. Radiology 1987; 164: 681–686

20 Jenkins JPR, Love HG, Foster CJ, Isherwood I, Rowlands DJ. Detection of coronary artery bypass graft patency as assessed by magnetic resonance imaging. Br J Radiol 1988; 61: 2–4

21 White RD, Pflugfelder PW, Lipton MJ, Higgins CB. Coronary artery bypass grafts: evaluation of patency with cine MR imaging. Am J Roentgenol 1988; 150: 1271–1274

22 Rzedzian R, Chapman B, Mansfield P, et al. Real-time nuclear magnetic resonance imaging in paediatrics. Lancet 1983; ii: 1281–1282

23 Stehling M, Chapman B, Glover P, et al. Real-time NMR imaging of coronary vessels. Lancet 1987; ii: 964–965

24 Pykett IL, Rzedzian RR. Instant images of the body by magnetic resonance. Magnetic Resonance in Medicine 1987; 5: 563–571

25 Rzedzian RR, Pykett IL. Instant images of the human heart using a new, whole-body MR imaging system. Am J Roentgenol 1987; 149: 245–250

26 Firmin DN, Klipstein RH, Hounsfield GN, Longmore DB. Echo-planar high resolution flow velocity mapping (Abstract). Berkeley: Society of Magnetic Resonance in Medicine, 1988; 7: 122

British Medical Bulletin (1989) Vol. 45, No. 4, pp. 968–990

MRI studies of atherosclerotic vascular disease: Structural evaluation and physiological measurements

R H Mohiaddin, D B Longmore
Magnetic Resonance Unit, The National Heart and Chest Hospitals

The widespread prevalence of atherosclerotic vascular disease has given rise to the need for a noninvasive imaging examination. Magnetic resonance imaging has been shown to allow assessment of early arterial disease non-invasively and without the use of ionising radiation. Arterial compliance, pulse wave velocity, and the pattern of flow within the aorta may all be disturbed by disease and these parameters can be measured by magnetic resonance. In addition, atheroma can be imaged directly, its size measured, its shape described, its lipid content assessed, and its effects upon vascular haemodynamics studied. Magnetic resonance imaging is thus a potential tool not only for the detection of disease but also for studying its natural history and the effects of interventions, such as the control of risk factors and of lipid lowering agents.

Atherosclerotic vascular disease is the commonest cause of death and disability in the western world.[1] Its pathogenesis is controversial[2] but the hypothesis that it is a response to injury, dating from the pioneering work of Virchow in 1856[3] and recently reviewed by Ross,[4] has gained widespread acceptance. A variety of lesions affect the arterial wall, from non-protruding fatty streaks to more complex lesions consisting of lipid, smooth muscle, fibro-

0007–1420/89/0045–0968/$10.00

blasts, and occasionally calcification. The morphology and composition of arterial segments containing atheroma is of considerable importance. Plaques of different morphology (concentric or eccentric, for example) have different effects on the arterial wall, such as the potential for thrombosis and the effect of arterial spasm.[5] The lipid content may also affect the propensity for fissuring, ulceration and thrombosis.[6] Other properties of atheroma that may be affected by the lipid content are the short and long term outcome of angioplasty, and the potential for regression.[7] Although little is known of these areas it is possible that there is a link between the composition of atheroma and its susceptibility to chemical or mechanical intervention. There is certainly evidence that regression can occur in experimental animals and that it may be possible to alter the rate of progression in man.[8]

Atherosclerosis leads to arterial stiffness both in experimental disease in animals[9] and in man,[10] and regression leads to reduced stiffness.[11] This mechanical alteration is a consequence of structural and biochemical changes and could well be a good index for the detection and monitoring of atherosclerosis at an early stage.

Magnetic resonance imaging provides a comprehensive assessment of atherosclerosis non invasively and without the use of ionising radiation. For instance, arterial compliance, pulse wave velocity, and the pattern of flow within the aorta may all be disturbed and these parameters can be measured by magnetic resonance. In addition, atheroma can be imaged directly, its size measured, its shape described, its lipid content assessed and its effects upon vascular haemodynamics studied. It is thus a potential tool not only for the detection of disease but also for studying its natural history, risk factors, and the effects of pharmacological or surgical interventions.

CHEMICAL SHIFT IMAGING OF ATHEROMA

Magnetic resonance has become an accepted imaging technique for the aorta and large vessels.[12,13] Because magnetic resonance signal is absent from flowing blood, high natural contrast exists between the lumen and the vessel wall, providing ideal circumstances for the demonstration of vascular anatomy and of atherosclerotic plaque. Conventional magnetic resonance imaging is able to demonstrate atheromatous lesions in *post mortem* human arteries, in experimental animal models, and in patients with atherosclerosis.[14,15] Most studies, however, have relied upon distortion of the arterial lumen and have not involved direct visualization of the atheroma. Those that have, have used conventional techniques which image hydrogen irrespective of chemical environment, and have not exploited the chemical shift of resonant frequency between the hydrogen in water and fat (3.3 parts per million). Imaging nuclei with only a particular resonant frequency rather than the entire spectrum of resonant frequencies is called chemical shift imaging.[16] Several techniques of proton chemical shift imaging have been described.[17] The method of Dixon[18] results in an image where pure water and pure fat produce no signal and tissues with a mixture of water and fat have higher signal (Fig. 1). The method of Hinks[19] is a true water or fat imaging technique where only signals from water or fat contribute to the image.

Figures 2 to 4 show applications of the Dixon technique. In Fig. 2, a raw egg is imaged. The subtraction image (Fig. 2B), which shows high signal from tissues with high concentration of lipid, shows high signal from the lipid rich yolk. Figure 3 shows a lipid rich atheromatous plaque in a *post mortem* human aorta. The in-phase magnetic resonance image shows both the plaque and an area of extravascular fat without information on lipid concentration, but the subtraction image shows that the plaque has a high lipid content. In contrast, Figure 4 shows a lipid deficient plaque with very low signal in the subtraction image (Fig. 4B). Figure 5 shows an example of the Hinks technique in a *post mortem* aortic specimen. High signal is seen in the extravascular fat but the lack of signal in the vessel wall indicates absence of lipid.

Patients with documented peripheral vascular disease have also been studied. Figure 6 shows an image of the descending abdominal aorta in which the circular lumen is distorted by thickening of the wall with an atheromatous plaque. The Dixon subtraction image shows that this plaque has low lipid content. Figure 7 shows another patient with a high lipid plaque.

MAGNETIC RESONANCE VELOCITY MAPPING

Magnetic resonance velocity mapping is described by Underwood in this Issue. Velocity profiles along an atheromatous vessel are particularly useful to localize disease and measure the degree of stenosis. Blood flowing into a stenosed region must accelerate and the mean velocity increase is proportional to the reduction of cross sectional area. Figure 8 shows anatomical images and velocity

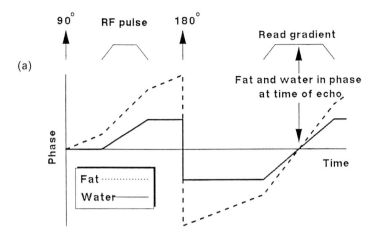

(a)

IN-PHASE SEQUENCE

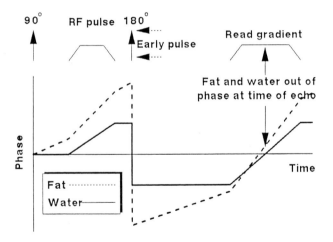

OUT OF PHASE SEQUENCE

Fig. 1a

maps of a normal abdominal aorta. The arterial wall is smooth and the velocity profiles through the aorta and iliac vessels are similar. Figure 9 shows images in a patient with peripheral vascular disease. The left iliac artery is narrowed and the velocity map shows high velocity past the obstruction. Figure 10 shows more extensive atheromatous disease involving the aortic bifurcation

(b)

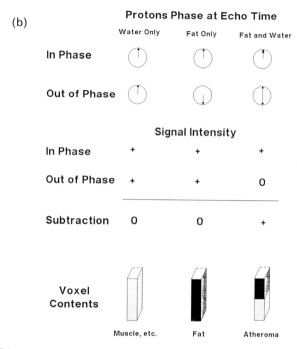

Fig. 1 Diagram of pulse sequences. (**a**) A conventional spin echo sequence with an echo time of 40ms gives an 'in phase' image because fat and water precess with the same phase at the time of the echo and the signal is the sum of that from fat and water. The second sequence is a modified asymmetrical spin echo sequence which gives an 'out of phase' image in which the signal is the difference of that from fat and water. (**b**) The phase of fat and water protons differs at the time of image acquisition in the 'in phase' and 'out of phase images'. Subtraction of the two images results in signal only from voxels containing both fat and water.

and the common iliac arteries. Figure 11 shows blood flow (L/min) at 16 points in the cardiac cycle (msec) in the abdominal aorta and common iliac arteries in a normal subject and in a patient with tight stenosis in his left iliac artery.

AORTIC COMPLIANCE

Compliance is the change in volume per unit change in pressure and it is a measure of stiffness and distensibility. The combination of elastic arteries and resistant arterioles constitutes a hydraulic filter enabling the intermittent cardiac output to be converted to a steady capillary flow. Part of the energy of left ventricular contraction produces forward flow during systole, but the remainder is

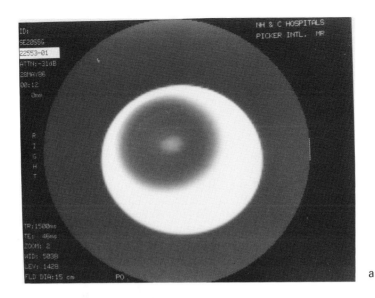

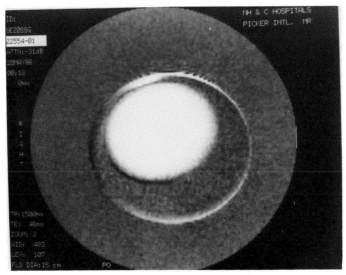

Fig. 2 (**a**) Conventional spin echo image of a raw egg shows high signal from both fat and water. (**b**) The subtraction image shows high signal in the lipid rich yolk.

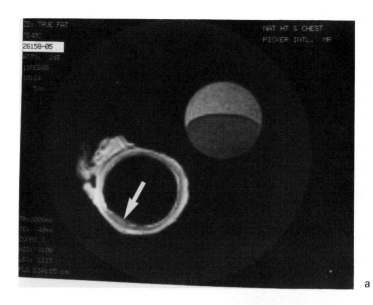

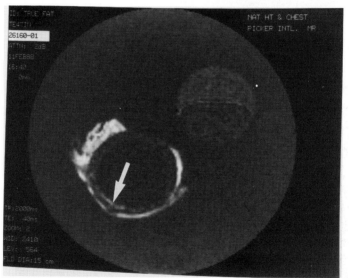

Fig. 3 (**a**) Post mortem aortic specimen imaged using a conventional spin echo sequence together with a phantom containing oil floating on water. Atheroma involves approximately half of the circumference of the vessel and the largest accumulation is arrowed. (**b**) The subtraction image shows high signal in extravascular fat and in the lesion. The ratio of signal intensity compared with extravascular fat is 45%. The oil and water in the phantom give low signal as expected.

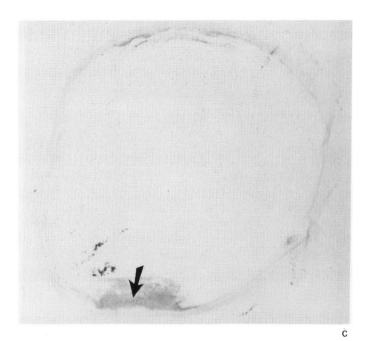

c

Fig. 3 (**c**) Histology of the same plaque (oil red O stain) showing lipid deposition within the intima (arrow).

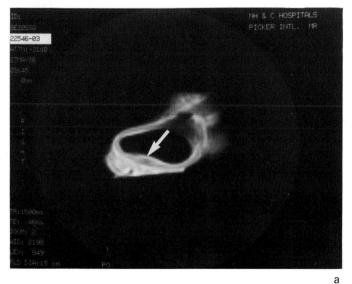

a

Fig. 4a

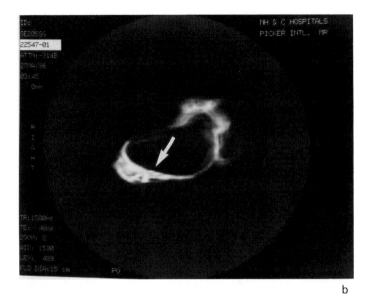

b

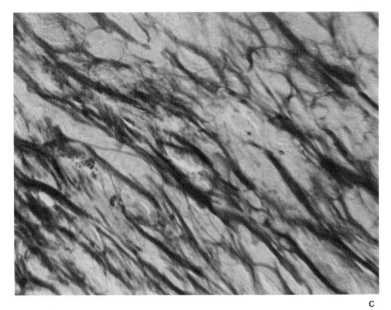

c

Fig. 4 (**a**) Conventional image of a lipid deficient plaque in a post mortem aortic specimen (arrowed). (**b**) The subtraction image shows very low signal (8%) compared with that from the extravascular fat. (**c**) Elastic Van Gieson stain (magenta) of the same plaque indicate a predominantly smooth muscle and fibrous plaque. Lipid deposition would appear as vacuoles in this alcohol treated stain, but there are none.

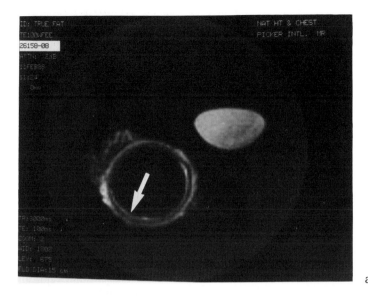

a

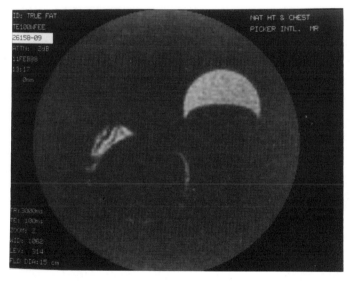

b

Fig. 5 True fat and true water images acquired using the Hinks technique. (**a**) In the water image, a *post mortem* aortic specimen lies beside a phantom containing oil floating upon water, but only the water is seen. The vessel wall is thickened by atheroma for 60% of its circumference (arrowed). (**b**) The fat image shows high signal from the extravascular fat, but low signal from the areas of atheroma, and in the phantom only the oil is seen.

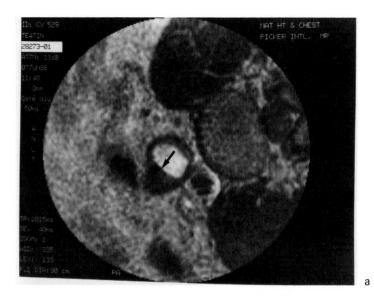

a

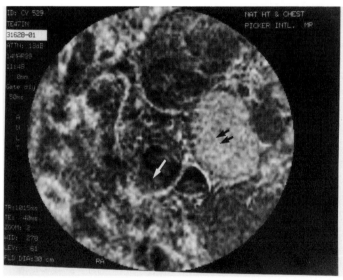

b

Fig. 6 (**a**) Spin echo image perpendicular to the descending aorta of a 60 year old man with peripheral vascular disease, showing a large atheromatous plaque expanding the vessel wall (arrowed). (**b**) The subtraction image shows low signal in the lesion (arrow) indicating low lipid content. There is high signal from extravascular fat and from the bone marrow in the body of the lumbar vertebra (double arrow).

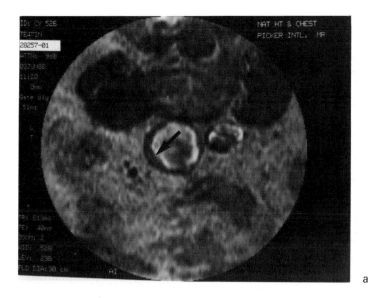

a

b

Fig. 7 (**a**) Spin echo image perpendicular to the descending aorta of a 57 year old man with peripheral vascular disease. The wall is irregularly thickened with atheroma and the main accumulation is arrowed. The subtraction image (**b**) shows high signal within the lesion indicating high lipid content (similar to the marrow in the lumbar vertebral body [double arrow]).

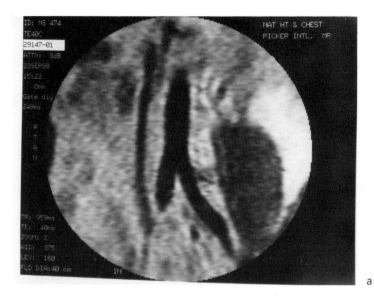

a

b

Fig. 8 (**a**) The aortic bifurcation anatomy in a normal 43 year old male. (**b**) The velocity in the aorta and both iliac arteries is the same.

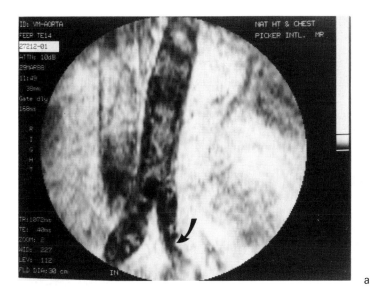

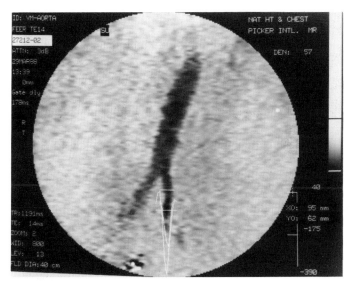

Fig. 9 (**a**) A 57 year old male with atheromatous disease. The left iliac artery is narrowed (arrow) on the anatomical spin echo image. (**b**) The velocity map shows high velocity profile past the obstruction.

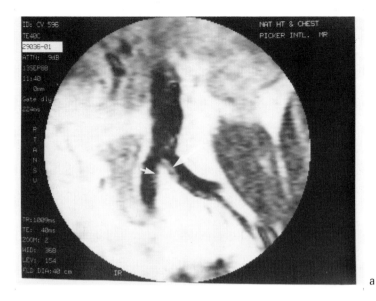

Fig. 10 (**a**) A 61 year old male with extensive atheroma at the bifurcation (arrows) demonstrated on the anatomical spin echo image. The velocity mapping image shows high velocity in the obstructed areas (**b**).

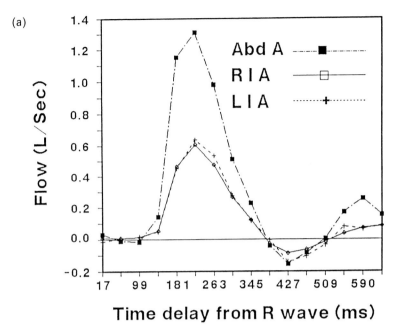

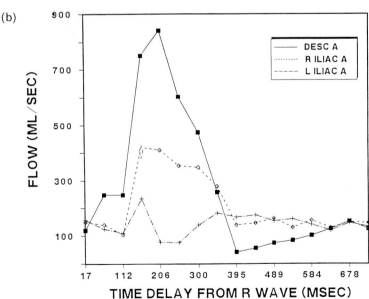

Fig. 11 Plot of flow values calculated from 16 frame velocity maps of the abdominal aorta, right and left common iliac arteries in a 36 year old healthy volunteer (**a**) and in a 50 year old male patient with tight stenosis in his left common iliac artery (**b**).

stored as potential energy in the distended arteries. During diastole, elastic recoil converts this potential energy into forward flow. A fall in aortic compliance increases the impedance to ventricular ejection and decreases capillary blood flow.[20,21] Aortic compliance, therefore, is a determinant of left ventricular afterload and it is important in patients with ventricular disease.[22]

Magnetic resonance imaging provides a direct noninvasive way of studying regional aortic compliance.[23] Images can be acquired at end diastole and end systole through the thoracic aorta (Fig. 12) and the change in volume between diastole and systole can be measured. The pulse pressure is measured using a conventional sphygmomanometer. In normal subjects, the ascending aorta is the most compliant region and compliance falls more distally. In athletes, regional aortic compliance is higher than normal, and in patients with coronary artery disease under the age of 50 it is lower (Fig. 13). These changes are likely to be the result of structural changes in the aorta and they are a potential screening tool for the detection of vascular disease.

AORTIC FLOW WAVE VELOCITY

The repeated ejection of the blood by the heart generates pressure and flow waves in the aorta and pulmonary artery, and these pulsations are transmitted throughout the arterial tree. The velocity of such waves depends principally on the distensibility and compliance of the vessel wall. If the vascular tree were rigid and the blood incompressible, the motion of blood in the root of aorta would be transmitted peripherally instantaneously. Blood is indeed incompressible, but the vessels are distensible in varying degrees, and the pulse wave velocity is finite.

Magnetic resonance provides a noninvasive method of measuring the flow wave velocity.[24] High temporal resolution (10 ms) velocity maps are acquired in a plane perpendicular to the ascending and descending aorta and the time taken for the flow wave to travel between the two points is measured (Fig. 14). Flow wave velocity increases with age (Fig. 15A) and with blood pressure and there is an inverse relationship between flow wave velocity and regional compliance (Fig. 15B). In the same way that aortic compliance may be used to detect vascular disease, flow wave velocity may also be a valuable parameter of the state of the arterial system.

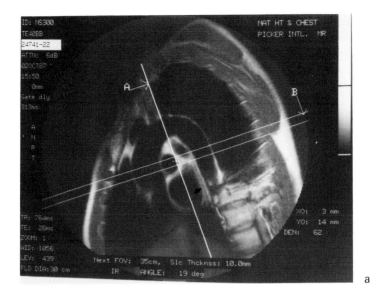

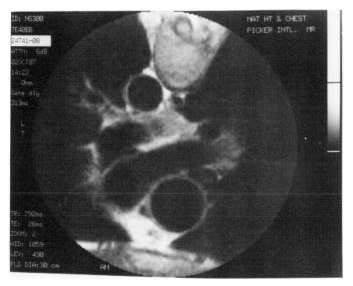

Fig. 12a and b

CONCLUSION

Although the application of magnetic resonance imaging to atheromatous vascular disease is in its early stages, the promise of a non-

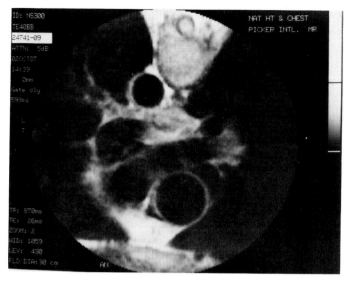

c

Fig. 12 (**a**) Oblique image of the ascending aorta, aortic arch and descending thoracic aorta illustrating the sites where compliance was measured. Diastolic (**b**) and systolic (**c**) images of the ascending and descending aorta showing the change in aortic area of a 38 year old normal volunteer.

Ascending aorta

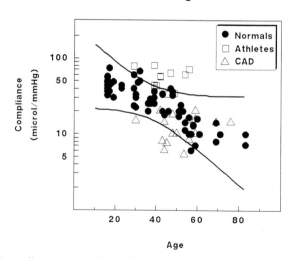

Fig. 13 Ascending aortic compliance displayed using a logarithmic scale and plotted against age. The regression equation is y = −0.01 × +1.79, and the 95% confidence intervals for the normal subjects are shown (r = −0.91, P < 0.001, SEE = 0.09). The figures of the athletes and patients with coronary artery disease are superimposed.

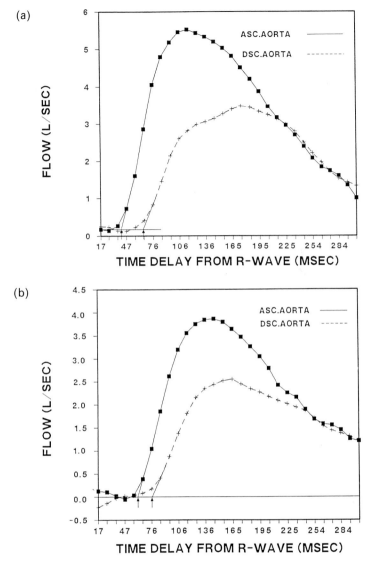

Fig. 14 The foot of the flow wave is defined by extrapolation of the rapid upstroke of the flow wave to the base line. The transit time needed for the flow wave to propagate from a point on the mid-ascending aorta and a point on the mid-descending thoracic aorta can be then calculated. (**a**) Data obtained from a young normal subject with good aortic compliance. (**b**) Data obtained from an elderly normal subject with poor compliance, the transit time is shorter than in the previous example.

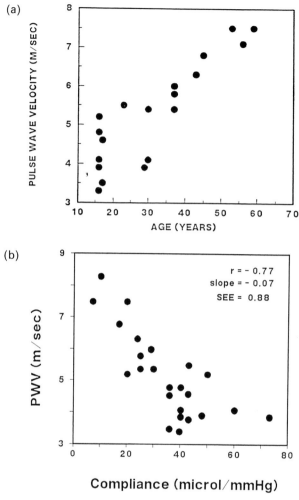

Fig. 15 The flow wave velocity is directly related to age (**a**), and is inversely related to regional aortic compliance (**b**).

invasive method for detecting disease and for assessing its structural significance promises to play an important role in the management of patients in the future.

ACKNOWLEDGEMENTS

We are grateful for the financial support of the Board of Governors of the National Heart & Chest Hospitals, the Coronary Artery Disease Research Association

(CORDA), and Picker International Ltd, and we should like to thank the staff of the magnetic resonance unit for their assistance.

REFERENCES

1 Report of the working group of arteriosclerosis of the National Heart, Lung and Blood Institute. Vol 2. Washington DC: Government printing office, 1981 [DHEW publication No.(NIH)82-2035]

2 Clarkson TB, Weingnad KW, Kaplan JR, Adams MR. Mechanisms of atherogenesis. Circulation 1987; 76: 1–20

3 Virchow R. Phlogose und thrombose im gefassystem, Gesammelte abhandlungen zur wissenschaftlichen medicin. Frankfurt-am-Main: Meidinger, 1856; p. 458

4 Ross R. The pathogenesis of atherosclerosis—an update. New Engl J Med 1986; 314: 488–500

5 Wissler RW, Vesselinovitch D, Davis HR, Lambert PH, Bekermeier M. A new way to look at atherosclerotic involvement of artery wall and the functional effects. Ann NY Acad Sci 1985; 454: 9–22

6 Smith E. Development of atherosclerotic plaque. In: Shillingford J, Birdwood G (eds). Impact of research on the practice of cardiology. London: British Heart Foundation, 1986; pp. 1–5

7 Potkin BN, Roberts WC. Effects of percutaneous transluminal coronary angioplasty on atherosclerotic plaques and relation of plaque composition and arterial size to outcome. Am J Cardiol 1988; 62: 41–50

8 Gotto AM. Regression of atherosclerosis. Am J Med 1983; 70: 989–91

9 Band W, Goedhard WJ, Knoop AA. Comparison of effects of high cholesterol intake on viscoelastic properties of the thoracic aorta in rats and rabbits. Atherosclerosis 1973; 18: 163–172

10 Banga I, Balo J. Elasticity of the vascular wall. 1 the elastic tensibility of the human carotid as a function of age and arteriosclerosis. Acta Physiol Acad Sci Hung 1961; 20–21: 237–247

11 Farrar DJ, Green HD, Wanger WD, Bond MG. Reduction in pulse wave velocity and improvement of aortic distensibility accompanying regression of atherosclerosis in Rhesus monkey. Circ Res 1980; 47: 425–432

12 Bogren HG, Underwood SR, Firmin DN, Mohiaddin RH, Klipstein RH, Rees RSO, Longmore DB. Magnetic resonance velocity mapping in aortic dissection. Br J Radiol 1988; 61: 456–4562

13 Glazer HG, Gutierrez FR, Levitt RG, Lee JKT, Murphy WA. The thoracic aorta studied by MR imaging. Radiology 1985; 157: 149–155

14 Herfkens R, Higgins C, Hericak H, et al. Nuclear magnetic resonance imaging of atherosclerotic disease. Radiology 1983; 148: 161–166

15 Wesby GE, Higgins CB, Amparo EG, Hale JD, Kaufman L, Pogany AC. Peripheral vascular disease: correlation of MR imaging and angiography. Radiology 1985; 156: 733–739

16 Pykett I, Rosen L. Nuclear magnetic resonance: in vivo proton chemical shift imaging. Radiology 1983; 149: 197–201

17 Brateman L. Chemical shift imaging: a review. Am J Roentgenol 1986; 146: 971–980

18 Dixon T. Simple proton spectroscopic imaging. Radiology 1984; 153: 189–194

19 Hinks RS, Quencer RM. Multislice chemical shift imaging by slice-selection gradient reversal. Magnetic Resonance Imaging 1988; 6: 22 (Abstract)

20 Berne RM, Levy MN. Cardiovascular Physiology. London: CV Mosby. 1981; pp. 94–97

21 Wilcken DE, Charlier AA, Hoffman JI, Guz A. Effect of alterations in aortic impedance on the performance of the ventricles. Circ Res 1964; 14: 283–293

22 Urschel CW, Covel JW, Sonnenblick EH, Ross J, Braunwald E. The effect of decreased aortic compliance on performance of the left ventricle. Am J Physiol 1968; 214: 298–304

23 Mohiaddin RH, Underwood SR, Bogren HB, et al. Regional aortic compliance studied by magnetic resonance imaging: The effects of age, training, and coronary artery disease. Br Heart J 1989; 62: 90–96

24 Mohiaddin RH, Firmin DN, Underwood SR, et al. Magnetic resonance measurements of aortic flow wave velocity: the effect of age and disease (Abstract). Berkeley: Society of Magnetic Resonance in Medicine, 1988; 7: 180

British Medical Bulletin (1989) Vol. 45, No. 4, pp. 991–1010
© The British Council 1989

Value of Ultrafast CT scanning in cardiology

M J Lipton[1]
W W Holt[2]
[1]*Department of Radiology and Medicine,* [2]*Departments of Medicine and Radiology,*
University of Chicago, Chicago, Illinois, USA

Computed tomography became available in 1973 and within a few years was accepted as a useful diagnostic technique in nearly every organ system. The heart, however, was the exception because long exposures (over 1 second) produced motion blurred images. Although ECG gating was possible it proved impractical. Conventional CT nevertheless has been undervalued by most radiologists and cardiologists who have little or no experience with cardiac CT. The recent development of Ultrafast CT should rapidly change this concept.[1]

ULTRAFAST CT SCANNER DESIGN AND OPERATION

The first high speed computed tomography scanner was developed at the Mayo Clinic.[2] This device, called the Dynamic Spatial Reconstructor (DSR), employs multiple X-ray tubes arranged in a circle around the patient which are fired in rapid sequence. This machine is one of a kind and has primarily been used as a research tool. More recently, Ultrafast CT (Imatron scanner C-100) developed by Douglas Boyd, is now available. This system is based upon electron beam technology, and, unlike conventional CT, this scanner has no moving parts except for the patient table. Several scanning options are currently available including almost simultaneous, multilevel, 50 ms scan acquisition at frame rates of up to 34 images per second (17 at each level). Two detector rings lie above the patient so that a pair of CT images are obtained each time any one of the tungsten rings is 'swept' by the electron beam, hence as many as eight levels can be scanned without table movement. Scans can be acquired at two, four, six or eight levels during a single acquisition. Slice thickness can also be varied from 3 mm to

0007–1420/89/0045–0991/$10.00

8 mm. Scanning is usually initiated from the patient's electrocardiogram and commences at a selected percentage of the cardiac cycle from 0–80% of the R-R interval: it can also be triggered manually. The specifications of the system are given in Table 1[1] and the scanning capability is summarized in Table 2.[1] The X-ray data once received at the detectors is converted to digital data. A powerful computer then reconstructs the images and displays them on a cathode ray oscilloscope. Further details of the Imatron C–100 scanner have been described elsewhere.[3,4]

ULTRAFAST CARDIAC CT SCANNING PROCEDURES

The basic scanning protocol is usually tailored to the clinical problem. However, in most patients, the following plan is generally followed. No premedications are given, and the patient fasts for at least four hours prior to examination. Standard ECG electrodes are placed on the patient's chest for continuous monitoring and for triggering the CT exposures. An 18-gauge, 5 cm long intravenous catheter is placed in either an antecubital vein or, when this is not possible, an external jugular vein. The CT table is then positioned to facilitate the acquisition of either short axis or long axis tomograms.[5] Table 3[1] identifies the indications for selecting these imaging planes. The mobile scanning platform allows the patient to be precisely tilted and slewed within the wide scanning gantry. Before contrast medium is given, localization scans are obtained and reviewed. The circulation time is assessed

Table 1 Cine-CT specifications

	Multi-level mode	Single-slice mode
Number of detectors/level	432	864
Number of levels per scan	2	1
Scan time	0.05 s	0.1–1.8 s (in 0.1 s steps)
Image matrix	256^3, 360^2	256^2, 360^2, 512^2
Slice thickness	8 mm	3 mm, 6 mm, 10 mm

Table 2 Cine-CT scanner capabilities

50 millisecond scan time for 2 sections
224 millisecond scan time for 8 sections
VOLUME MODE: reconstruction in any plane
CINE MODE: 2 simultaneous levels; 17 frames/s
FLOW MODE: time vs. density or area profiles
HIGH RESOLUTION MODE: 100 millisecond scan time

Table 3 Indications for ultrafast CT in long and short cardiac axes

Long axis	Short axis
Simultaneous imaging of all four cardiac chambers	Simultaneous evaluation of anterior, lateral, posterior, and interventricular septal surfaces of left ventricle.
Atrioventricular valve function	Quantitation of left ventricular mass
Evaluation of left ventricular apex for thrombi or tumor	Evaluation of the aorta and aortic valve
Evaluation of pericardial disease (thickening, effusion, calcification)	Quantitation of segmental left ventricular function
Quantitation of the extent of left ventricular apical and posterior/basal aneurysms	Evaluation of the extent of left ventricular posterior aneurysm
Evaluation of global and regional left ventricular function	Evaluation of atrial septal defect
Evaluation of septal defects	Quantitation of global right and left ventricular volumes
Evaluation of bypass graft patency	
Characterization of arrythmic foci	

by noting deflection time from an ear oximeter following an intravenous bolus injection of 0.2 mg indocyanine green dye. Contrast medium is administered using a flow controlled injector (Medrad Co., Pittsburgh) and for quantitative CT studies a non-ionic agent is essential and injected at between 3–7 ml/second. The patient is requested to suspend respiration for a few seconds before and during scanning at a comfortable mid or maximal inspiratory level. This level should be constant for all subsequent series. Most cooperative patients manage this quite well. Scanning is usually performed to obtain coverage of all ventricular levels in both the flow and movie acquisition modes (Table 2).

DATA ANALYSES

All images are reviewed level by level. Image analysis is performed using a variety of operator-interactive programs. These allow accurate placement using a track ball guided cursor of cardiac chamber borders as well as quantitations of tomographic wall thickness, chamber volumes and function. Digital imaging allows precise quantitation of CT data. There are essentially two general approaches for evaluating cardiac anatomy and function; one is based upon measurements of motion and the other on measurements of flow. These techniques will now be described to illustrate some typical clinical applications of Ultrafast CT.

CARDIAC BORDER DEFINITION AND LEFT VENTRICULAR MASS

It is essential that proper cardiac border (edge) definition and placement be assured for quantitation of left ventricular anatomy and function. A quantitative method of cardiac edge detection for Ultrafast-CT was developed initially for the determination of left ventricular mass by Skioldebrand et al.[6] and was applied to Ultrafast-CT by Feiring et al.[7] This technique, which is a direct application of principles originally used for transmission X-ray devices nearly 30 years ago, defines the absolute placement of the cardiac edge at a CT density (Hounsfield scale) halfway between the density of the myocardium and adjacent structures. This requires evaluation of the CT density of the left and right ventricular cavities, the anterior chest wall, lung and adjacent myocardium.

Placement of the endocardial and epicardial surfaces, as a direct and straightforward application of this 'full width/half maximum' method noted above, is aided by an operator defined, computer assisted, semi-automated edge definition program included in the standard Ultrafast-CT data analysis software. The operator determines the placement of the cardiac edge by defining the center of the CT number density (level) and range of CT densities (window) that constitute the density of the endocardial or epicardial surfaces. The software then outlines the contour and determines the absolute value of area within. Minor vagaries in computer aided placement of the cardiac edge can be corrected by the operator using a tract-ball device. Global measurements of left ventricular mass and volumes are performed at the data analysis console or workstation following definition of left ventricular endocardial and epicardial contours at each level from apex to aortic root.

As an initial application of this method of border definition and validation of the quantitative potential of Ultrafast-CT, a study of left ventricular mass was performed in 22 consecutive dogs.[7] Short axis tomograms from left ventricular apex to aortic root were acquired in the volume mode during suspended respiration following a slow infusion of iodinated contrast. Following completion of each study the absolute left ventricular mass was then determined by direct measurement on a standard laboratory scale.

Subsequently, end-diastolic scans were evaluated from cardiac apex to base using the border definition method noted above. Calculation of left ventricular mass was made using the modified Simpson's rule and knowledge of the scanning target geometry by subtracting the endocardial volume from the epicardial volume and multiplying by the myocardial density. Comparison between left ventricular mass *in situ* and that calculated by Ultrafast-CT in vivo is shown in Figure 1.[7] The correlation is excellent ($r = 0.99$) and the standard error of the estimate on the order of 4.1 g. Additionally, inter- and intra-observer variability has been assessed and the technique found to be highly reproducible.

Left ventricular mass has been measured by fast CT and 2-D echocardiography in a small series of patients and correlated reasonably well as shown in Figure 2.[8]

CALCULATION OF LEFT AND RIGHT VENTRICULAR VOLUMES

Reiter et al.[9] performed a study in dogs assessing the determination of left ventricular stroke volume by Ultrafast-CT compared with that derived simultaneously using either a chronically im-

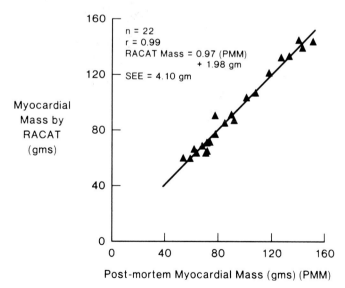

Fig. 1 Comparison of absolute postmortem myocardical mass of the canine left ventricle with in vivo determination using ultrafast computer tomography. (Reproduced by permission of Circulation, Ref. 7.)

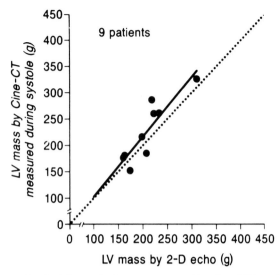

Fig. 2 Regression for left ventricular mass measured by cine-CT (systolic images) and calculation by 2-D echo. (Reproduced by permission of Radiology, Ref. 8.)

planted and calibrated aortic electromagnetic flow probe or careful assessment using established thermodilution techniques. Electro-cardiographically triggered scans were acquired in the movie mode nearly simultaneously from the cardiac apex through the base in the short axis during intravenous slow injection of iodinated contrast. Stroke volume was then calculated as the difference between end-diastolic (peak of R wave) and end-systolic (smallest cavity) volumes again, using direct application of Simpson's Rule. Stroke volume has been determined by Ultrafast-CT ($r = 0.99$, slope-1.01, SEE-1.5 ml) even in the presence of acute myocardial infarction.[9] If left ventricular stroke volume can be quantitated by Ultrafast-CT then, by inference, determinations of end-diastolic and end-systolic volume should be, likewise, quantitative. Studies done using casts of canine left ventricles have previously shown the accuracy of static estimates of left ventricular volume by conventional CT.[10]

Simultaneous determination of right ventricular volumes is possible with the determinations of left ventricular mass and volumes. As an addition to the studies of left ventricular volume noted above, Reiter et al. also determined right ventricular stroke volumes[9] by planimetry of the tomographic volumes of the end-diastolic and end-systolic scans and re-applying Simpson's Rule. Application of this method then makes no assumptions as to right (or left) ventricular geometry as is commonly used for contrast angiography.[11] Calculated right ventricular stroke volume compared absolutely with the left ventricular stroke volumes. As with the left ventricular volume calculations, inter- and intra-observer variability was minimal. The direct measurement of right ventricular (RV) volume by CT is expected based upon studies of RV casts.[12]

In conclusion, Ultrafast-CT can be used to provide highly quantitative data regarding left and right ventricular volumes provided careful attention is paid to proper border definition. Direct application of these data to a normal population has recently been reported.[13,14]

INTERVENTIONAL ULTRAFAST CT

Because scan acquisition is so fast and no ECG gating is required, the use of interventions is possible in conjunction with Ultrafast CT scanning.

A number of centers are using bicycle ergometer exercise for quantitative studies of left ventricular ejection fraction and regional wall motion abnormalities.[15] Caputo et al. compared radionuclide exercise studies with fast CT in one patient subgroup.[16] Exercise is feasible with cine-CT and should complement isotope studies in that CT can measure regional wall thickening dynamics (not possible with radionuclide methods) by virtue of its high spatial and temporal resolution as shown in Figure 3A and B.[1] Ultrafast CT procedures can also be successfully performed in conjunction with cardiac pacing electrode interventions.

More recently attention has focussed on studies of the right ventricle with ultrafast CT. Echocardiography has difficulties with this chamber while CT displays it well and Cine-CT can be recommended for most forms of right ventricular dysfunction.[17]

CARDIAC ANATOMY AND PATHOLOGY

One of the attributes of Ultrafast-CT scanning is the exquisite detail with which cardiac anatomy can be defined. This coupled with the ability to determine global and regional function provides a firm basis from which one can evaluate cardiac anatomy.

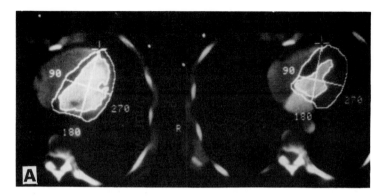

Fig. 3A One level from a multilevel sequence of ultrafast-CT scan depicting normal contraction at rest—the endocardial and epicardial boundaries have been outlined for endiastole and endsystole at rest. (Reproduced with permission of Cardiology Clinics, Ref. 1.)

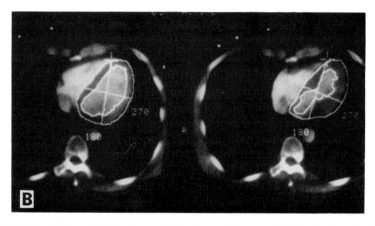

Fig. 3B The same level as shown in 3A above, during exercise showing impaired regional wall contraction in the anterioseptal zones. Note the distortion of the left ventricular cavity compared with the normal appearance as seen at rest in 3A. (Reproduced with permission of Cardiology Clinics, Ref. 1.)

CORONARY ARTERIES

As CT technology advances, image resolution improves. Figure 4 illustrates a typical scan through the aortic root showing proximal portions of the coronary arteries. Calcification is detected readily in these vessels with great clarity using fast CT. In this particular respect, cine-CT is unique and has the potential to be a useful screening procedure. One series, in a selected population

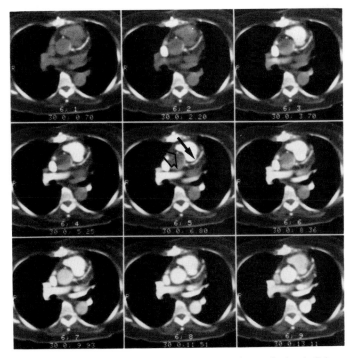

Fig. 4 Typical ultrafast-CT scan, with contrast, imaging at the level of the aortic root. Calcified proximal portions of the left (solid arrow) and right (open arrow) coronary arteries are clearly seen. The frames depict cardiac events proceeding from end-diastole (upper left frame) through systole (lower right frame).

undergoing coronary arteriography, found that calcification was predictive in high risk patients and detected calcification in the coronary arteries in more patients than fluoroscopy. CT detected all the positive fluoroscopy studies.[18]

The addition of the high resolution (100 ms) volumetric scanning capability to the high temporal resolution (50 ms) cine and flow mode scanning allows for combined studies which use the advantages of both methods of scan acquisition. One such example is the evaluation of constrictive pericardial disease. Although standard CT can be used to evaluate pericardial thickening, this has previously been used only as an anatomical tool with relationship to cardiac function determined by two-dimensional echocardiography and/or invasive cine-angiography. Combined use of the 100 ms mode to provide high spatial resolution tomography for determination of pericardial thickening has recently been combined with high temporal resolution scanning to provide physiological information in patients with clinically suspected constrictive pericardial disease.[19]

Many of the manifestations of ischaemic heart disease can be determined non-invasively by two-dimensional echocardiography and/or radionuclide angiography; however, definition of the extent of left ventricular aneurysms is difficult with these methods and is only partly answered with the use of invasive cine-angiography. Ultrafast-CT promises to provide highly detailed examinations of left ventricular aneurysms, regardless of anatomic location.

Recent studies by Reiter et al.[20] document the ability of Ultrafast-CT to quantitate regurgitant volumes. Additional studies by Rumberger et al. using Ultrafast-CT[21] have also demonstrated that details of left ventricular diastolic function may be derived in such patients which may allow for additional characterization of the physiological load placed on the cardiac muscle, independent of the regurgitant volume.

CHARACTERIZATION OF LEFT VENTRICULAR DIASTOLIC FUNCTION

Early diastolic filling of the left ventricle is an active, energy dependent process that is distinct from systolic emptying. Several cardiac pathological states have been identified where abnormalities in early diastolic function dominate over the clinical presentation. Routine characterization of left ventricular diastolic dynamics is emerging as a useful clinical tool usually evaluated via two-dimensional echocardiography/mitral Doppler velocimetry[22] or radionuclide equilibrium angiography.[23] However, limited acoustic windows and the assessment of only global mitral inflow characteristics reduce the extension of ultrasound studies to all patients. Radionuclide angiography is probably the most widely described technique to evaluate details of left ventricular filling, but the low spatial resolution and the non-tomographic aspect of the images limit additional information as to absolute volumes and details of ventricular anatomy and myocardial wall dynamics.

Ultrafast-CT examinations in the movie or 'cine' mode provide high temporal and spatial resolution tomographic information through the cardiac cycle at multiple left ventricular levels which is amenable to calculations of left ventricular filling characteristics on a global (Simpson's Rule) and regional (tomographic) basis. Images are generally acquired at four to six adjacent left ventricular levels in the cardiac short axis with up to 20 images/level. Triggering on the R wave of the ECG then allows for up to approximately 1200 ms of tomographic time dependent data which is sufficient to scan through all of systole and into the period of diastasis for all patients in normal sinus rhythm with heart rates greater than 40/min. An example of a raw, unsmoothed time dependent left ventricular tomographic volume data is shown on Figure 5. Note the classic features of end-diastole, rapid systolic emptying, end-systole, rapid diastolic filling, diastasis and the atrial systole.

Characteristics (global and tomographic) of the rapid filling phase are determined using methods previously employed in radionuclide angiography.[24] Basically the volumetric data from end-systole, through rapid filling and into the initial portion of diastasis is fit to a third order polynomial (sigmoid shape) and the absolute peak rate of filling, time to peak filling from end-systole and the fraction of total filling occurring at the time of peak filling (filling fraction) is determined directly from the curve fit data.

Studies in 11 normal patients employing Ultrafast-CT have been previously reported.[25] In this group of normal subjects global peak filling rate (PFR) (sum of six contiguous tomographic scan series) was normalized to end-diastolic volume (EDV) to allow for ready horizontal comparison to data available from the literature using standard radionuclide angiographic methods. In

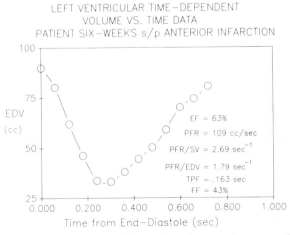

Fig. 5 Example of time dependent left ventricular volume changes throughout the cardiac cycle at the midventricle in a normal patient. (Reproduced by permission of the Journal of the American College of Cardiology.)

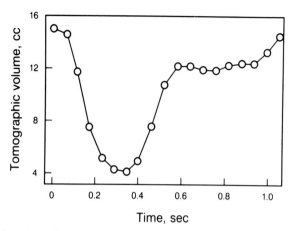

Fig. 6 Time-dependent left ventricular volume curve as a mean of 6 contiguous left ventricular tomographic slices. Note that the character of the left ventricular volume curve during early filling is distinctly different from that seen in the normal patient in Figure 5. (Reproduced by permission of the Journal of the American College of Cardiology, in press.)

these subjects the normalized peak filling rate (PFR/EDV) was 3.15 ± 0.15 s.$^{-1}$ This value is in total agreement with data in normals reported from several prior studies.[23,24,26]

The above data then form a basis for characterization of early diastolic filling data in patients with a variety of cardiac diseases. An example from a patient six weeks after an initial Q-wave anterior wall myocardial infarction is shown on Figure 6. Despite a normal ejection fraction and stroke volume, the absolute peak rate of filling and normalized peak filling rates (using both end-diastolic volume, EDV and stroke volume, SV) are significantly reduced. The time to peak filling (TPF) is moderately delayed but the filling fraction (FF) is normal.

Ultrafast CT is an emerging imaging modality that has been shown to be highly applicable to quantitative determinations of ventricular mass, right and left ventricular volumes and global and regional left ventricular function in a variety of cardiac pathological states. The attractiveness of Ultrafast-CT lies not so much on a single determination of diastolic filling in a given individual, but on the strength of easily acquired, highly reproducible and accurate serial imaging in patients following pharmacological or interventional therapy directed at abnormalities in early diastolic filling.

CORONARY ARTERY BYPASS GRAFT PATENCY

This application was the first cardiac CT procedure to gain acceptance. Patency is recognized when there is contrast enhancement of the grafts coincident or just following peak enhancement of the ascending aorta. CT is particularly valuable in the early postoperative period. This is because the surrounding fat is radiolucent and highlights the contrast enhanced grafts dramatically. All levels—as many as eight—can be scanned during one injection of contrast agent and during the same held inspiration. Because relatively little contrast medium is required Cine-CT allows routine studies of the left ventricle during the same procedure. A multicenter trial compared ultrafast CT to arteriographic assessment of graft patency in 127 grafts (saphenous and internal mammary). Results showed a sensitivity of 93%, specificity of 89% and an accuracy of 92% (Fig. 7).[27] Analysis of the time-density curves generated by the CT computer for grafts and the aorta allows assessment of graft flows using peak arrival times before and after dipyridamole. A study of this technique in dogs has been reported by Rumberger et al.[28] Studies of flow rates and flow reserve, before and after intravenous dipyridamole, are very encouraging in patients for determining graft quality.

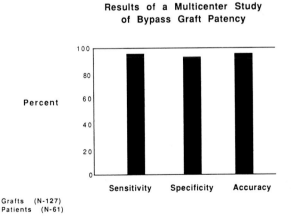

Fig. 7 Sensitivity, specificity and predictive accuracy of evaluating bypass grafts with ultrafast computed tomography in Group I. (Reproduced by permission from JACC. Ref. 27.)

MEASUREMENTS OF BLOOD FLOW

No present imaging modality can measure regional myocardial blood flow in absolute terms with any degree of precision. Radioactive microsphere measurements in animals constitute the best available laboratory method known and require sacrificing the animal. Thallium-201 imaging in man provides useful but, nonetheless, only relative estimates of regional myocardial perfusion. Nearly all our techniques for evaluating ischemic heart disease are, in fact, indirect, including coronary arteriography and left ventriculography.

Blood flow measurements that are to be clinically useful may be considered in two groups: (a) blood flow through the cardiac chambers and vessels such as the carotid arteries and coronary bypass grafts and (b) blood flow measurements in tissue, which are much more difficult.

Cardiac output has been measured and validated by cine-CT.[29] The accuracy of cine-CT was validated against simultaneous thermodilution measurements of cardiac output, and the results showed excellent correlation ($r = 0.92$) with the mean percentage of difference between these techniques being 9.7% over a range of 1.5 to 6.3 liters per minute.[29]

The ability to obtain a bimodal time-density curve over any cardiac chamber or vascular region involved in left-to-right or right-to-left shunting provides a measure of the size of the shunt.[30]

MYOCARDIAL PERFUSION

The diagnosis and therapy of patients with ischaemic heart disease would be benefitted by the availability of a routine, safe, reliable and minimally invasive means to quantitate regional myocardial perfusion. Perhaps the most important application of such a method would be in the determination of the physiological significance of coronary artery stenoses. It is clear that the clinical interpretation of coronary angiograms is variable given the diffuse nature of coronary disease in man[31] and more solid physiological information is provided by the assessment of coronary/myocardial flow reserve.[32] However, recent reviews on the concept of coronary/myocardial flow reserve point to some of the shortcomings of this approach alone[33] and underlie the additional need for **absolute** determinations of myocardial flow rates as well. Ultrafast

Computed Tomography offers an approach which may provide not only determinations of relative flow and flow reserve between various cardiac regions, but also provides for quantitation of regional flow per unit mass to virtually any cardiac region.

By means of electrocardiographically triggered exposures at a designated time during the cardiac cycle (nominally one scan every other QRS), stop action images can be obtained using Ultrafast-CT as iodinated contrast (vascular indicator) traverses the left ventricular cavity, proximal aorta and myocardium. Available off-line image analysis software allows for characterization of arterial (input) and myocardial (response) indicator transit curves within any operator defined region of interest within the tomogram. The application of Ultrafast-CT to the determination of tissue perfusion relies on direct application of classical indicator dilution theory.[28,34]

Derivations directly from classical indicator dilution theory[35] allow for definition of a basic algorithm for determination of regional flow (perfusion) per unit mass of myocardium. This is calculated directly from derived characteristics of contrast clearance curves within the left ventricular cavity (or aorta) and myocardium without the need for additional parameter scaling or referencing. An equation identical to that derived by Axel[36] for determination of cerebral perfusion using CT and that employed by Mullani et al.[37] for positron emission studies of myocardial perfusion using ^{82}Ru can be applied.

IN VITRO AND IN VIVO STUDIES

Jaschke et al.[38] performed a phantom study using Ultrafast-CT where a system of tubes was employed to simulate vessels and a central cylinder packed with small, irregularly shaped plastic parts used to simulate a tissue equivalent.

Wolfkiel et al.[39] performed a study of regional myocardial perfusion using Ultrafast-CT in 16 dogs employing femoral vein injection of contrast under control, vasodilated and ischaemic conditions. Their results are shown in Figure 8. Note in particular that the calculation of regional flow per unit mass is linear under ischemic and control conditions up to values of approximately 150 ml/100 g/min; above this range the calculation by CT seriously underestimated the actual flow; in fact, the calculation reaches a 'plateau' at the higher flow rates.

A recent study by Gould, Lipton and colleagues[40] attempted to

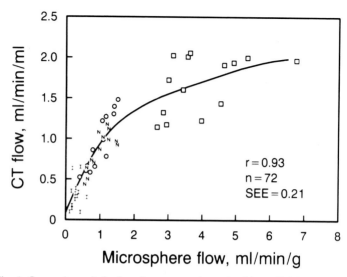

Fig. 8 Comparison of absolute flow rate as determined by radiolabelled micros-pheres vs. CT calculations of regional myocardial perfusion. (Reproduced by permission of the American Heart Association, Ref. 39.)

account for the potential 'plateau' of the CT calculations at high flow rates using intravenous contrast medium injection and mod-ifying the basic flow algorithm. Addition of this factor could allow for the first order deconvolution between the input and the response. This algorithm could allow extension of the calculation by Ultrafast-CT using intravenous injection techniques across the physiological range, Plate 11. At normal flows and up to twice normal flows, however, there was an excellent correlation. This suggests that Ultrafast-CT may be very useful in the clinical setting for estimating regions of myocardial ischaemia.[40]

A further explanation of the underestimation of CT calculations at higher flow rates can be provided, at least partly, by the recent studies of Wan et al.[41] using the Dynamic Spatial Reconstructor at the Mayo Clinic (a prototype high speed three-dimensional CT device). They reported calculations of regional perfusion by CT, linear up to 800 ml/100 g/min using aortic root injection of contrast in lieu of intravenous injection. This observation suggests that the coronary input function (bolus) kinetics are of prime importance for the CT technique to be successfully applied over the entire dynamic range for values of regional myocardial perfu-sion. This underscores the limitations of the theoretical approach with specific considerations to assumptions[35] including the assumption that the indicator input can be considered to be instantaneous, and of the clinical usefulness of the CT method. However, recent developments into a further understanding of regional myocardial vascular blood volume[42] suggest that this is a dynamic parameter, which, if excluded from analysis may contribute more importantly to the underestimation noted by Rumberger[34] and Wolfkiel[39] at high flow rates, than does complex considerations of venous versus systemic injection bolus kinetics.

In summary, the application of Ultrafast-CT techniques to the quantitation of regional myocardial perfusion is an evolving process where it is clear that limitations are multifactoral. A limitation remains regarding input function kinetics if the entire dynamic range of possible regional myocardial perfusion is to be studied. However, use of the less invasive intravenous injection method over a more invasive and clinically impractical systemic injection method may be worthwhile for a given subject. The data presented from the study by Rumberger et al.[34] employing an inferior vena cava injection has recently been re-evaluated in lieu of dynamic changes in regional myocardial vascular volume[42] where preliminary studies now suggest that regional perfusion can be quantitated up to 400 ml/100 g/min. If normal resting flow is approximately 100 ml/100 g/min,[43] this would imply that studies could be done with intravenous injection methods in order to characterize regional myocardial perfusion flow reserve up to a ratio of 4:1. Values above this would be underestimated. However, studies by Wilson, et al.,[44,45] using a unique intracoronary Doppler catheter, have shown that 'normal' flow reserve (in the absence of hypertrophy) is 3.7:1 or greater and that patients with physiologically significant coronary artery disease have a reserve of usually less than 3:1.

CONCLUSIONS

Computed tomography represents the optimal theoretical approach to X-ray imaging. This conclusion arises from its capacity to solve the fundamental limitation of all forms of X-ray imaging, that is, the superimposition of anatomic structures. Because CT is a fully three-dimensional method, this problem is addressed in a manner not subject to the risks, complications and technical limitations of selective angiography, subtraction angiography, tomography, and many other techniques. Therefore, the optimism for cine-CT imaging of the heart is well founded. Apart from the demonstration of anatomic structures in any plane and in real time in movie format, this new generation of CT scanners offers a unique potential for measuring myocardial perfusion. This can be evaluated in two ways: by measuring myocardial wall thickening, which is a sensitive indicator of blood flow, and by assessing time-density changes due to the passage of contrast agent through thin slices of myocardium. Neither of these techniques can be performed adequately at present with noninvasive or even invasive techniques. Feasibility studies, however, have demonstrated that this should indeed be possible using fast CT scanning. The radiation exposure of current whole-body scanners is low.[46] The radiation exposure to the patient with the cine-CT scanners is comparable to or less than that with the whole body scanner; hence, this will not be a practical limitation.

Obviously, further controlled clinical studies are needed to validate the capability of Ultrafast-CT for general clinical purposes, and comparisons will be necessary with established angiographic, echocardiographic, and nuclear medicine techniques. Further studies are also needed in animals as well as patients to determine the sensitivity and specificity of Cine-CT. Should Ultrafast-CT reach its anticipated potential, electron-beam systems of this type may not only replace present third- and fourth-generation CT scanners for general whole body purposes, but also Ultrafast-CT may become a complementary or even the primary screening and diagnostic cardiac imaging technique of the future.

REFERENCES

1 Rumberger JA, Lipton MJ. Ultrafast cardiac CT scanning. In: Wolfe CL, ed. Cardiology Clinics. Philadelphia: Saunders 1989 (In press)

2 Ritman EL, Robb RA, Johnson SA, et al. Quantitative imaging of the structure and function of the heart, lungs and circulation. Mayo Clin Proc 1978; 53: 3–11

3 Boyd DP, Gould RG, Quinn JR, et al. A proposed dynamic cardiac 3D densitometer for early detection and evaluation of heart disease. IEEE Trans Nucl Sci 1979; 26: 2724–2727

4 Peschmann KR, Couch JL, Parker DL. New developments in digital X-ray detections. SPIE Proc 1981; 314: 5054

5 Rees MR, Feiring AJ, Rumberger JA, et al. Heart evaluation by cine CT: use of two new oblique views. Radiology 1986; 159: 805

6 Skioldebrand CG, Lipton MJ, Mavroudis C, et al. Determination of left ventricular mass by computed tomography. Am J Cardiol 1982; 49: 63–70

7 Feiring AJ, Rumberger JA, Reiter SJ, et al. Determination of left ventricular mass in the dog with rapid acquisition cardiac CT scanning. Circulation 1985; 72: 1355

8 Diethelm L, Simonsen JS, Dery R, et al. Measurement of LV mass by ultrafast CT and 2-D echocardiography. Radiology 1989; 171: 213–217

9 Reiter SJ, Rumberger JA, Feiring AJ, et al. Precision of measurements of right and left ventricular volume by cine computed tomography. Circulation 1986; 74: 890–900

10 Lipton MJ, Hayashi TT, Boyd D, et al. Measurement of left ventricular cast volume by computed tomography. Radiology 1978; 127: 419–424

11 Dodge HT, Hay RE, Sandler H. An angiocardiographic method for directly determining left ventricular stroke volume in man. Circulation 1962; 11: 739

12 Ringertz HG, Rodgers B, Lipton MJ, et al. Assessment of human right ventricular cast volume by CT and angiocardiography. Invest Radiol 1985; 20: 29–32

13 Feiring AJ, Rumberger JA, Reiter SJ, et al. Sectional and segmental variability of left ventricular function: Experimental and clinical studies using ultrafast computed tomography. JACC 1988; 12: 415–425

14 Stark CA, Rumberger JA, Reiter SJ, et al. Use of cine CT in assessing the severity of aortic regurgitation in patients,. Circulation 1986; Suppl. II-4 Abstract. 74

15 Lipton MJ, Rumberger JA. Exercise ultrafast computed tomography: Preliminary findings on its role in diagnosis and prognosis of coronary artery disease. Editorial comment. JACC 1989; 13(5): 1082–1084

16 Caputo GR, Gould R, Dery R, et al. Cine CT evaluation of exercise induced ischemia: A feasibility study. Dyn. Cardiovasc. Imag., in press.

17 Himmelman RB, Abbott JA, Lipton MJ, Schiller NB. Cine computed tomography compared with echocardiography in the evaluation of cardiac function in emphysema. Am J Card Imag 1988; 2(4): 283–291

18 Reinmuller R, Lipton MJ. Detection of coronary artery calcification by computed tomography. Dyn Cardiovasc Imag 1987; 1(2): 139–145

19 Sheedy PF, McCusik MA, Rumberger JA, et al. Fast CT evaluation of patients with possible constrictive pericarditis. 74th Session of the Radiology Society of North America, Chicago, Illinois, USA, 1988

20 Reiter SJ, Rumberger JA, Stanford W, et al. Quantitative determination of aortic regurgitant volumes by cine computed tomography. Circulation 1987; 76: 728–735

21 Rumberger JA, Vonk GN, Sinak LJ, et al. Impaired early diastolic filling in patients with compensated aortic insufficiency. Circulation 1988; 78: II–399

22 Rokey R, Kuo LC, Zoghvi WA, et al. Determination of parameters of left ventricular diastolic filling with pulse doppler echocardiography: Comparison with angiography. Circulation 1985; 71: 543

23 Pollak JF, Kemper AJ, Bianco JA, et al. Resting early peak diastolic filling rate. A sensitive index of myocardial dysfunction in patients with coronary artery disease. J Nucl Med 1982; 23: 471–478

24 Reduto LA, Wickemeyer WJ, Young JB, et al. Left ventricular diastolic performance at rest and during exercise in patients with coronary artery disease. Circulation 1981; 63: 1228–1237

25 Rumberger JA, Stark CA, Stanford W, et al. Heterogeneity of diastolic filling in normal patients as assessed by cine computed tomography. JACC 1987; 9A: 159

26 Miller TR, Goldman KJ, Sampathkumaron KS, et al. Analysis of cardiac diastolic function: Application in coronary artery disease. J Nucl Med 1983; 24: 2–7

27 Stanford W, Brundage BH, MacMillan R, et al. Sensitivity and specificity of assessing coronary bypass graft patency with ultrafast computed tomography: Results of a multicenter study. JACC 1988; 12(1): 1–7

28 Rumberger JA, Feiring AJ, Hiratzka LF, et al. Quantitation of coronary artery bypass flow reserve in dogs using cine computed tomography. Circ Res 1987; 61 (suppl 2): 117–123

29 Garrett JS, Lanzer P, Jaschke W, et al. Measurement of cardiac output by cine computed tomography. Am J Cardiol 1985; 56: 657–661
30 Garrett JS, Jaschke W, Aherne T, Botvinick EH, Higgins CB, Lipton MJ. Quantitation of intracardiac shunts by Cine-CT. JCAT 1988; 12(1): 82–87
31 Arnett EN, Isner JM, Redwood DR, et al. Coronary artery narrowing in coronary heart disease: comparison of cine angiographic and necropsy findings. Ann Intern Med 19   ; 91: 350–6
32 White CW, Wright CB, Doty DB, et al. Does the visual interpretation of the coronary arteriogram predict the physiologic significance of a coronary stenosis? N Eng J Med 1984; 310: 819–824
33 Klocke FJ. Measurements of coronary flow reserve: Defining pathophysiology vs. making decisions about patient care. Circulation 1987; 76: 1183–1189
34 Rumberger JA, Feiring AJ, Lipton MJ, et al. Use of ultrafast CT to quantitate myocardial perfusion: a preliminary report. JACC 1987; 9: 59–69
35 Zierler KR. A simplified explanation of the theory of indicator-dilution for measurement of fluid flow and volume and other distributive phenomena. Bull John's Hopkin's Hosp 1958; 103: 199
36 Axel L. Cerebral blood flow determination by rapid sequence computed tomography: theoretical analysis. Radiology 1980; 137: 679–86
37 Mullani N, Goldstein RA, Gould KL, et al. Myocardial perfusion with rubidium–82. II. Measurements of extraction fraction and flow with external detectors. J Nucl Med 1983; 24: 898–906
38 Jaschke W, Gould RH, Assimakopoulos PA, et al. Flow measurements with a high speed computed tomography scanner. Med Phys 1987; 14(2): 238–243
39 Wolfkiel CJ, Fergson JL, Chomka EF, et al. Measurement of myocardial blood flow by ultrafast computed tomography. Circulation 1987; 76: 1262–1273
40 Gould RG, Lipton MJ, McNamara MT, et al. Measurement of regional myocardial blood flow in dogs by ultrafast CT. Invest Radiol 1988; 23: 348–353
41 Wan T, Wu X, Chung N, et al. Myocardial blood flow quantitated by synchronous, multislice, high speed computed tomography. IEEE Trans Med Imag 1989 (In press)
42 Rumberger JA, Bell MR, Sheedy PF, et al. In vivo quantitation of intramyocardial blood volume by ultrafast computed tomography. Circulation 1988; 78: II–398
43 Rumberger JA, Stanford W, Marcus ML. Quantitation of regional myocardial perfusion by ultrafast computed tomography: promises and pitfalls. Am J Card Imag 1987; 1,4: 336–343
44 Wilson RF, Laughlin DE, Ackell PH. Transluminal subselective measurement of coronary blood flow velocity and vasodilator reserve in man. Circulation 1985; 72: 82–92
45 Wilson RF, Laughlin DE, Hartley CB, et al. Selective measurements of coronary blood flow velocity and vasodilator reserve in man. JACC 1984; 3: 529
46 Brasch RC, Boyd DP, Gooding CA. Computed tomography scanning in children: Comparison of radiation dose and resolving power of commercial CT scanners. AJR 1978; 131: 95

British Medical Bulletin (1989) Vol. 45, No. 4, pp. 1011–1035
© The British Council 1989

Echocardiography of valve disease

P Wilde
Department of Radiodiagnosis, Bristol Royal Infirmary, Bristol, UK

Recent technical developments have led to the combined use of imaging and Doppler modalities in cardiac diagnosis to produce a reliable and non-invasive approach to the accurate assessment of cardiac valve disease. Anatomical detail is visible on two dimensional imaging, accurate measurement and timing can be derived from M-mode studies and Doppler studies give detailed insight into cardiac valve haemodynamics. In the majority of patients valve gradients can be calculated using continuous wave Doppler techniques, while pulsed Doppler techniques (including colour flow mapping) can give accurate information about valve regurgitation. In many cases these techniques provide an adequate substitute for cardiac catheterisation and they can be repeated as often as necessary to monitor progress of disease and treatment.

The echocardiographic assessment of cardiac valve disease has advanced in the last decade to a position where a virtually complete evaluation of all cardiac valves is possible in the majority of patients. This is due to the development of high resolution two dimensional (2D) echocardiography[1] using phased array or mechanical sector scanners and more recently the introduction of Doppler techniques. Many of the Doppler capabilities are incorporated into imaging instruments so that precise flow patterns can be determined within the heart at specific sites.[2] Some instruments will incorporate colour flow mapping and this can be most useful although, at present, it is not generally regarded as essential in the diagnosis and quantitation of cardiac valve disease. As familiarity with colour flow mapping grows it is becoming increasingly useful in making examinations faster and more accurate.

Historically M-mode scanning was the precursor to 2D and Doppler echocardiography but M-mode techniques are no longer

0007–1420/89/0045–1011/$10.00

the main part of a cardiac ultrasound examination. The 2D should now be the 'core' of the examination and from this the basic cardiac anatomy and much of the pathology will be identifiable. This will be particularly so if full use is made of all the echocardiographic windows available on the chest. M-mode and Doppler evaluation will be selected to make certain specific measurements of structure or function as deemed appropriate by the clinical indication and the findings on 2D examination. M-mode examination will therefore be used in any patient where left ventricular function is being studied because it provides an accurate method of calculating the changing diameter across any part of the ventricle. This should, however, not be taken in isolation but should be incorporated with the overall appearance of the left ventricle seen on 2D echocardiography.

Fast moving structures, particularly associated with cardiac valves, may be more easily recorded by M-mode studies and the technique may also be used for recording the precise timing of events, occasionally with a simultaneous phonocardiogram. Once a particular flow abnormality is suspected, either from clinical or preceeding imaging findings, it will be necessary to use Doppler flow measurements to determine the more precise nature of these flow abnormalities.

In general terms, pulsed wave Doppler will be used for precise sampling within different parts of the heart to determine the site, direction, velocity, intensity and character of flow. In some cases high velocities will not be recordable by pulsed techniques due to the physical limitations of the technique. In this situation the continuous wave transducer will be used to measure the high velocity. Colour flow mapping will often highlight abnormal or unusual flows, particularly when they occur in unexpected directions.

Echocardiography has the advantage over clinical examinations in that each separate cardiac valve can be examined separately and thus complex abnormalities can be resolved stage by stage. The ultrasound techniques will often produce haemodynamic data of equivalent or better quality than can be produced at catheterisation, but it is important to become familiar in practice with the strengths and weaknesses of the two approaches.

Stenotic valves can often be assessed by measuring the flow velocity in the jet of blood passing through the stenosis. In the case of a given flow (e.g. a normal cardiac output) an increasingly narrow orifice or stenosis will lead to an increasingly high velocity of flow through that orifice. The Bernoulli equation has been modified for use in cardiac patients and in its most simple form is represented as:

$$P = 4\,V^2$$

Where P = pressure drop across the stenosis (mmHg) and V = velocity (m/s)

This simplified version of the equation makes the assumption that true velocity has been recorded (i.e. the Doppler interrogation beam is in line with flow) and that the blood velocity before the stenosis (i.e. in a cardiac chamber) was negligible. This calculation can be easily applied to determine the peak instantaneous gradient across any valve. It can also be used to calculate the mean gradient during the flow period and it can be used to determine the pressure differential between two chambers in the case of a regurgitant valve. Full details of these methods have been described elsewhere.[3]

Absolute volume flow at a point in the circulation can be calculated if the mean velocity of flow is known at that point and the cross-sectional area at that point is also known (usually from echocardiographic imaging data).

$$\text{Volume flow (ml/s)} = \text{Mean Velocity (cm/s)} \times \text{Area (cm}^2)$$

This principle can be used in theory to determine the flow at any point in the cardiac circulation but it has been difficult to apply and can only be used if particular techniques are established. Cardiac output can be measured from the ascending aorta if accurate Doppler measurements are taken from the same point as an accurate cross sectional measurement of the left ventricular outflow tract or aortic view.

There are methods whereby volume flow studies can be used to measure the regurgitant fraction through abnormal cardiac valves but they are generally time consuming and require meticulous technique if accurate results are to be obtained.

Individual valve lesions will be discussed below in terms of qualitative diagnosis, quantitation and additional findings.

MITRAL STENOSIS

Qualitative diagnosis of mitral stenosis

Mitral stenosis is a condition in which there is usually a rheumatic aetiology which produces thickening of the valve leaflets and

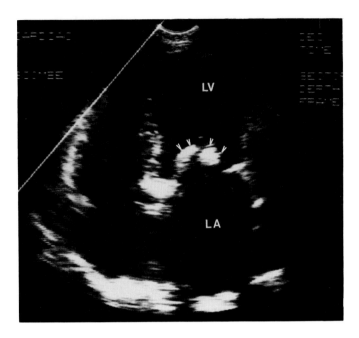

Fig. 1 Apical four chamber view showing mitral stenosis. The heavily echogenic leaflets (arrowed) dome in diastole and have a small central orifice (left ventricle—LV, left atrium—LA).

fusion of the commissures which thus restricts the orifice size. This means that the normal opening of the valve is restricted and a characteristic dome shape is seen during diastole with a central small orifice visible on the 2D image (Fig. 1). In addition there may be thickening and fusion of the chordae tendineae. An additional M-mode feature to confirm the diagnosis is a loss of the normal opposite motion of anterior and posterior leaflets, which in severe mitral stenosis tend to move almost together due to the marked commissural fusion. The thickening of the leaflets may become intense and echogenic due to calcification within the tissues.

With the addition of Doppler techniques, mitral stenosis becomes particularly easy to diagnose. The traditional methods of evaluating the mitral valve by the M-mode technique have largely given way to Doppler evaluation. Normal flow through the mitral valve takes place in two phases which can clearly be recognized on a Doppler recording (Fig. 2). The initial passive flow in early diastole is produced because the ventricle relaxes completely and

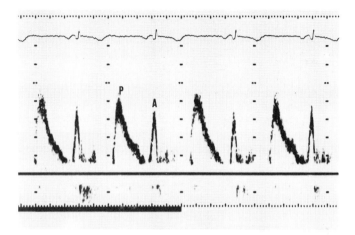

Fig. 2 Apical pulsed Doppler recording of normal mitral flow. Passive early diastolic flow (P) and active atrial induced flow (A) are seen in each cycle.

allows flow from the slightly higher pressure left atrium. This flow normally takes place very quickly and there is typically a mid-diastolic reduction or cessation of flow before a second phase of flow caused by atrial systole. In the case of mitral stenosis the initial flow persists at relatively high velocity because the narrow orifice of the valve cannot immediately relieve the pressure differential between the atrium and the ventricle. Thus a high velocity flow is produced by the pressure gradient and this only gradually decreases as the pressure gradient between the two chambers is released. In addition the normal smooth (laminar) flow through the widely open valve becomes a narrow turbulent jet through the stenotic orifice. These features are clearly recognized on the spectral trace as well as being clearly distinct on the audio channel of the instrument. On colour flow examination the narrow high velocity jet through a stenotic mitral valve is clearly recognizable.

Mitral stenosis can also be caused in the elderly patient by thickening of the leaflets due to annular fibrosis and calcification. This is much less common than rheumatic stenosis and a considerable degree of annular thickening is required to produce any significant degree of mitral obstruction.

In some patients with a dilated left ventricle, the mitral annulus will be stretched and this can give an apparent dome shape to the open valve in diastole. This must not be confused with mitral stenosis and can clearly be differentiated because the leaflet tips move well and the mitral orifice size is normal.

Quantitation of mitral stenosis

Traditionally the M-mode trace has been used to measure the diastolic closure rate of the mitral valve, this parameter having an approximate inverse correlation with the severity of stenosis. Two dimensional imaging can be used with moderate reliability to measure the orifice size of a stenotic mitral valve. The approach to quantitation of mitral stenosis has, however, radically changed since the introduction of Doppler evaluation.

The severity of mitral stenosis can easily be determined if a good quality trace is obtained in line with the direction of flow through the valve. This is usually possible from at or near the cardiac apex. The shape of the flow envelope on the spectral trace can be used to determine:[4]

1. The peak gradient
2. The end diastolic gradient
3. The mean gradient
4. The pressure half time.

The most useful gradient measurement is probably the mean gradient but this value is relatively dependent on the length of the cardiac cycle and the degree of activity of the patient. The mitral pressure half time has proved to be a highly useful indicator of the severity of mitral stenosis.[5] It is based on the principle that the pressure gradient between atrium and ventricle is relieved quickly by a normal valve and increasingly slowly by more severely stenotic valves. The time taken for the initial pressure gradient to drop to half its original level can be calculated in milliseconds and this has been shown to correlate well with the valve orifice size (Fig. 3). This parameter is much less dependent on heart rate and exercise level than the pressure gradient across the mitral valve.

Additional findings in mitral stenosis

Mitral stenosis has a profound effect on the size of the left atrium. In most cases there is significant atrial enlargement and in longstanding examples of this disease the left atrium can become massively enlarged (Fig. 4). In some circumstances there will be thrombus formation within the stagnant blood in the left atrium

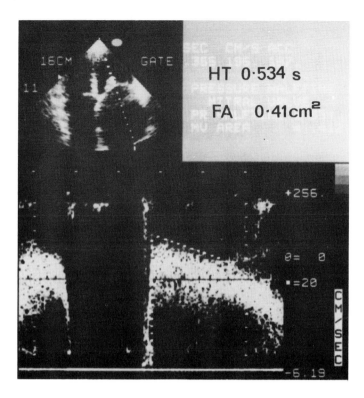

Fig. 3 The small inset shows a pulsed Doppler beam aligned with a stenotic mitral valve from the apex. The spectral trace shows the slow decrease in velocity seen typically in sevee mitral stenosis. The pressure half time (HT) and functional valve area (FA) have been calculated.

and this will often be detectable on 2D imaging. In cases of severe mitral stenosis the left ventricle will remain rather small due to the reduced flow of blood into it and the left ventricular contractility will be normal, as judged on the M-mode or 2D echocardiogram.

Mitral stenosis will raise the pulmonary venous pressure and this in turn will raise pressures on the right side of the heart. In chronic examples there may be pulmonary hypertension with dilatation of the pulmonary artery, right ventricle, and right atrium. This dilatation will often produce secondary effects of pulmonary and tricuspid regurgitation. Pulmonary hypertension may also be present. This can often be indicated by the raised jet velocity through the regurgitant tricuspid or pulmonary valves. Associated aortic valve disease is often seen and occasionally tricuspid stenosis is seen in chronic rheumatic heart disease.

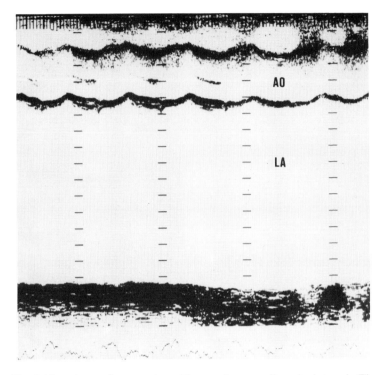

Fig. 4 M-mode trace from a patient with severe long-standing mitral stenosis. The grossly enlarged left atrium (LA) is 11 cm in diameter. It lies behind the aortic root (AO).

A stenotic mitral valve may become infected but small vegetations will be very difficult to see in the presence of a thickened and irregular valve. Only large mobile vegetations can be clearly seen.

MITRAL REGURGITATION

Qualitative diagnosis of mitral regurgitation

Mitral regurgitation can be very difficult to diagnose on imaging studies alone. In a limited number of cases there will be obvious pathology which must be associated with regurgitation, for example ruptured chordae which lead to a flail mitral leaflet moving back into the left atrium during ventricular systole. Mitral valve prolapse is more difficult and is not always associated with regurgitation. Many cases of mitral regurgitation are not associated with any visible abnormality of the mitral valve. Mild mitral regurgitation is a common finding in cases of dilated or abnormally functioning left ventricle and varying degrees of mitral regurgitation are associated with mitral valve stenosis. Infective endocarditis is often associated with mitral regurgitation and mitral valve vegetations can certainly be taken as a clue to the presence of mitral regurgitation.

Mitral regurgitation can however only be detected with confidence by the use of Doppler techniques.[6] The precise positioning of a pulsed Doppler sample volume behind the closed leaflets of a mitral valve will reveal a high velocity turbulent flow in systole indicating regurgitation. This abnormal flow will clearly be demonstrated on colour mapping and the distribution of the jet in the left atrium can be determined by pulsed Doppler mapping or colour flow mapping (Plate 12). It is very important to examine the entire left atrium to determine the direction of flow of the regurgitant jet. Continuous wave Doppler studies can also clearly demonstrate mitral regurgitation (Fig. 5). It is important when using non-imaging techniques (usually continuous wave) not to confuse mitral regurgitation and aortic stenosis. In an apical examination both these abnormalities will produce a high velocity systolic flow away from the transducer. The easiest way to distinguish the two is by appropriate movement of the transducer, separately recognizing the aortic and mitral regions. If this is not possible then identification will be feasible by assessment of the overall flow velocities and the timing of the various flows. The movement of the mitral and aortic valves will often produce artefacts on a Doppler trace which can be used to differentiate the two flows.

Quantitation of mitral regurgitation

The main approach to quantitation of mitral regurgitation has been the use of Doppler echocardiography and jet mapping. The distribution of the regurgitant jet in the left atrium together with its overall intensity is the best guide to the severity of mitral regurgitation. This is somewhat analogous to the approach used in assessing mitral regurgitation in angiography and with either approach accurate quantitation is difficult. Pulsed Doppler examination can be used to map the left atrium carefully using access from all echo windows and using all planes. In this way a full 3D assessment can be achieved. If colour flow mapping is available, a similar form of assessment can be carried out more quickly.[7]

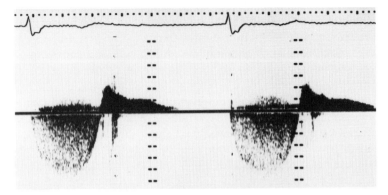

Fig. 5 Apical continuous wave Doppler recording in a patient with mitral regurgitation. Normal diastolic flow is shown above the baseline and the high velocity regurgitant jet is seen below the baseline (peak velocity 5.4 m/s). The patient also has a bradycardia.

Current Doppler systems are capable of detecting very minor degrees of mitral regurgitation and it is important to develop a good level of understanding of the sensitivity of any instrument being used to avoid over emphasizing the importance of this lesion.

The absolute jet velocity in mitral regurgitation is unhelpful in the assessment of severity of the lesion because there is always a large pressure differential between the left ventricle and the left atrium. A jet of mitral regurgitation in the presence of severe aortic stenosis will probably produce the highest of all velocities in the human circulation. If a patient with a normal blood pressure (120 mmHg in systole) and a severe aortic valve gradient (for example, 140 mmHg) then the overall left ventricular systolic pressure will be 260 mmHg. This may produce a jet of approximately 8 metres/second. This does not necessarily mean that the volume of regurgitant blood is large.

Additional findings in mitral regurgitation

Haemodynamically significant mitral regurgitation will cause volume overloading of the left ventricle which will normally show increased cavity size and increased stroke volume. The left atrium may be enlarged also, particularly if this is a chronic condition and if associated with rheumatic mitral stenosis. Acute severe mitral regurgitation (e.g. due to a ruptured chordae tendineae) is often associated with a normal sized left atrium. There will also be right sided cardiac effects which can be similar to those seen in mitral stenosis.

AORTIC STENOSIS

Qualitative diagnosis of aortic stenosis

In the majority of cases of aortic stenosis seen in adult patients there is considerable thickening of the aortic valve leaflets together with restricted mobility. In late cases, the leaflets become intensely echogenic due to the calcification within them. The commonest cause of isolated aortic stenosis in adults is the progressive stenosis of a congenitally previously bicuspid aortic valve. Aortic stenosis associated with rheumatic heart disease is also found but is less common and is usually associated with other valve disease. In the case of congenital aortic stenosis the valve leaflets may be thin, flexible and mobile but show doming in systole. The thickening of aortic leaflets and the restricted mobility are clearly seen on M-mode traces. Two dimensional echocardiography will confirm this as well as demonstrating the presence of a bicuspid valve, if this is present. The orifice area of the aortic valve can be measured but this is somewhat inaccurate due to the irregular orifice and the artefacts produced when scanning such an intensely echogenic structure.

Doppler studies will clearly reveal the presence of aortic stenosis if the high velocity jet through the stenotic lesion is recorded. This can be done from the cardiac apex, the subcostal position, the right parasternal or the suprasternal position. In most situations is it easier to use the 'pencil beam' of the continuous wave transducer rather than the localized sample volume of pulsed Doppler system. In the latter situation the depth of the aortic valve will also make pulsed Doppler less helpful because 'aliasing' of the high velocity signal will occur.

It is important in cases of aortic stenosis to search for and exclude other related lesions namely, sub-aortic stenosis (fixed or dynamic) and supra-aortic stenosis.

Quantitation of aortic stenosis

The quantitation of aortic stenosis is based on the recording of the frequency shift produced by the high velocity jet passing through the aortic valve and determining the velocity of flow from this.[8]

Accurate recording must be made in a direction close to that of the aortic jet. A number of different windows may be tried to get the optimal signal. Once the peak jet is recorded the modified Bernoulli formula can be used to calculate the gradient across the valve (Fig. 6). Analysis of the flow envelope will permit measurement of the peak instantaneous gradient as well as the mean gradient.

It is important to differentiate peak instantaneous gradient from the typical gradient across the aortic valve measured by a catheter pull back technique. In the latter situation the pressure in the left ventricle and aorta are not recorded simultaneously so that the peak pressures in the two chambers will often be occurring at different times. Thus the so called 'peak to peak' catheter method can give a result lower than obtained by peak instantaneous recording. When analysing any discrepancy between Doppler and catheter measurements it is important to consider the possibility of this technical difference which can cause an apparent overestimate of the gradient by Doppler examination. Doppler examination can also underestimate a gradient if the ultrasound beam is placed

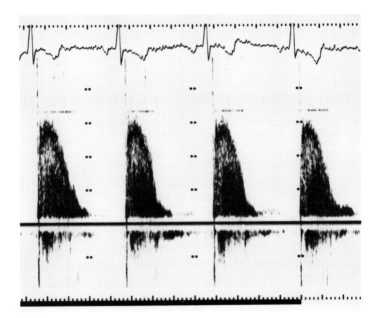

Fig. 6 Suprasternal continuous wave Doppler recording in a patient with moderately severe aortic stenosis. The peak velocity is 3 m/s which indicates a peak instantaneous gradient of 36 mmHg.

inappropriately at a large angle to the direction of flow through the valve.

In some patients with poor left ventricular function the cardiac output will drop. In this case the pressure gradient across the aortic valve will also drop but this is a true phenomenon and this will occur whether the pressure gradient is measured at catheter or by Doppler techniques.

Additional findings in aortic stenosis

In longstanding cases of aortic stenosis there will be hypertrophy of the left ventricular walls with good contractility and a normal chamber size. In very longstanding cases there can be deterioration of left ventricular function with enlargement of the cavity and poor overall contractility. The ascending aorta will often be dilated due to the post stenotic effects. Associated right sided cardiac changes are less common than with mitral valve disease except in the late stages of left ventricular failure. There can be infected vegetations on a stenotic valve but these are often difficult to see in the presence of prominent echoes from the valve leaflets.

AORTIC REGURGITATION

Qualitative diagnosis of aortic regurgitation

Aortic regurgitation is difficult to detect accurately on imaging techniques alone. Secondary effects may be obvious in some cases; for example fine fast vibration of the anterior leaflet of the mitral valve may be caused by the jet of aortic regurgitation and this can sometimes be recorded on M-mode tracings.[9] Left ventricular cavity size and wall motion may be altered by volume overload and, of course, specific pathology affecting the aortic valve itself may be identified. In the latter case vegetations or prolapse of the aortic valve may be seen and will often indicate the presence of regurgitation (Fig. 7).

Doppler studies are the most sensitive way of detecting aortic regurgitation and indeed they are probably the most accurate method of all, even surpassing angiography in mild regurgitation. A pulsed Doppler sample volume placed immediately beneath the aortic valve will reveal a high velocity jet of turbulent flow in any case of aortic regurgitation. Pulsed Doppler studies will often show this to be aliasing and continuous wave examination is needed to record the peak velocity which is likely to be high due

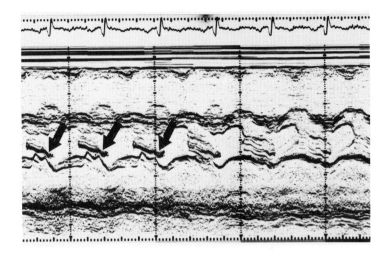

Fig. 7 M-mode trace sweeping from the left ventricular outflow tract (left of trace) to the aortic valve (right of trace). A large aortic vegetation is seen prolapsing into the outflow tract in diastole (arrowed). This was associated with aortic regurgitation.

to the large pressure differential between the aorta and left ventricle in diastole. Colour flow Doppler will clearly reveal a jet of aortic regurgitation (Plate 13) and this has the advantage that the size and direction of the jet can clearly be identified and jet mapping is rather more straightforward than with pulsed Doppler which is more time consuming.

Quantitative evaluation of aortic regurgitation

As with mitral regurgitation jet mapping using Doppler techniques has been the most frequently used method of ultrasonic quantitation.[10] This is somewhat subjective however, as it relies on good technique and consistency of interpretation to ensure good differentiation between different grades of regurgitation. There are however, other useful additional approaches to the assessment of severity. Continuous wave tracings of the aortic regurgitant jet will show a characteristic envelope shape.[11] If the pressure gradient remains high throughout diastole, this indicates a persisting high differential between aorta and left ventricle and therefore is more likely to be found in mild aortic regurgitation (Fig. 8). If the velocity of the regurgitant jet decreases throughout diastole this indicates a lower pressure differential between aorta and left

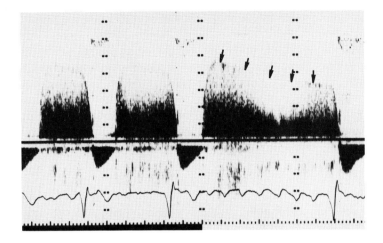

Fig. 8 Apical continuous wave Doppler trace taken from a patient with mild aortic regurgitation. The high velocity but low intensity jet of diastolic aortic regurgitation above the baseline shows only slight reduction in velocity during diastole (arrowed).

ventricle in late diastole. This in turn suggests severe regurgitation with possible raised left ventricular filling pressure. Another approach to the assessment of severity of aortic regurgitation is measurement of the reverse flow component in the aortic arch.[12] A suprasternal pulsed wave approach to the upper descending aorta can be made in most patients and this allows good alignment of the ultrasound beam with flow directions. In normal patients there is only a transient reversal of flow in the aorta in early diastole but with progressively increasing severity of regurgitation, there is a larger and larger reverse flow component visible (Fig. 9). The combination of the three approaches described above will usually give a very adequate assessment of severity of aortic regurgitation.

Additional findings in aortic regurgitation

Chronic aortic regurgitation can often be tolerated well for long periods and the left ventricle usually dilates somewhat to compensate for the leak through the valve and the consequent volume overload. The left ventricle therefore shows increased contractility with a dilated cavity. In late cases the left ventricle may show damage and become poorly contractile. The wall may be hypertrophied but this is not usually as marked as with aortic stenosis. The dilatation of the left ventricle may produce some mitral regurgitation due to annular dilatation but this is usually mild and not of clinical importance. Individual pathological processes will often be seen in association with the aortic regurgitation, aortic root aneurysm or annuloaortic ectasia being common findings in association with severe aortic regurgitation. Occasionally dissection of the ascending aorta is a cause of the regurgitation. The aortic regurgitation found in association with aortic stenosis is usually less significant than the stenosis, although occasionally it can be severe.

TRICUSPID VALVE

The principles of examination of the tricuspid valve are essentially the same as those used for evaluation of the mitral valve. The tricuspid orifice is somewhat larger than the mitral orifice and in addition to this the pressure gradients in the right side of the heart causing normal flow are lower than those on the left and thus the Doppler flow patterns show lower velocity even than seen in a normal mitral valve. Tricuspid stenosis is a relatively unusual

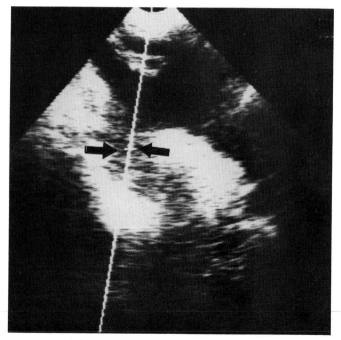

Fig. 9 (a)

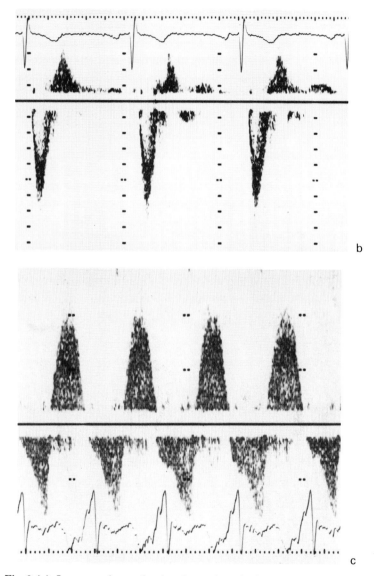

b

c

Fig. 9 **(a)** Suprasternal scan showing the aortic arch. A pulsed Doppler sample volume is placed in the upper descending aorta (arrowed). **(b)** Pulsed Doppler trace recorded from the position shown in (a) in a patient with mild aortic regurgitation. Normal systolic flow down the descending aorta is shown below the baseline and is followed by a low velocity reverse flow component that persists throughout diastole. **(c)** Continuous wave Doppler trace from a similar position as shown in (a) from another patient. The reverse flow component is larger than in (b) and indicates aortic regurgitation of more severe degree than in (b).

accompaniment of rheumatic heart disease but when present can clearly be diagnosed on a Doppler trace. In addition the gradient assessment in tricuspid stenosis is often as reliable as that obtained at catheterisation where many difficulties are encountered in assessment of tricuspid valve disease.

Tricuspid regurgitation is a much more common finding[13] and in fact mild or trivial tricuspid regurgitation can be found in many normal people. In patients with significant left sided cardiac disease there is often secondary tricuspid regurgitation due to some right ventricular dilatation. If this is present it can be used to advantage because continuous wave Doppler techniques can be used to measure the peak jet velocity from right ventricle to right atrium. This in turn can be used to measure the pressure differential between these two chambers in systole. If the right atrial pressure is known either by direct measurement or by clinical estimation, then this can be added to the right ventricular to right atrial pressure differential to give an estimate of pulmonary artery pressure (right ventricular pressure is similar to pulmonary artery pressure assuming no pulmonary stenosis).

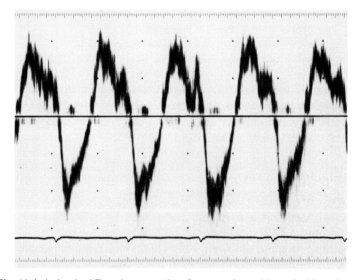

Fig. 10 Apical pulsed Doppler trace taken from a patient with carcinoid syndrome and severe tricuspid regurgitation. The sample volume is placed in the valve orifice. There is a very large systolic component of regurgitation shown below the baseline. The velocity of the normal diastolic flow towards the transducer (above the baseline) is increased due to severe volume overload.

In a few patients there may be organic disease confined to the tricuspid valve, either of infective origin or due to the carcinoid syndrome (Fig. 10).

PULMONARY VALVE

The pulmonary valve is relatively infrequently a cause of problems in the adult population. Occasionally with sensitive Doppler equipment pulmonary regurgitation is detected and this is becoming more apparent as the use of colour flow techniques increases. Pulmonary regurgitation is a recognized finding in a minority of the normal population. This jet can also be used to determine pressure differentials and the pulmonary diastolic pressure can sometimes be estimated from this reverse flow.

Stenosis of the pulmonary valve can be evaluated with imaging and Doppler studies in much the same way as the aortic valve. It is important to remember the possibility of infundibular (muscular) pulmonary stenosis which can occur just below the pulmonary valve. The peak velocity of flow through the pulmonary valve must therefore be compared with that immediately proximal to the valve. In this way a sequential gradient may be determined.

PROSTHETIC CARDIAC VALVES

Non invasive ultrasound studies are particularly valuable in the assessment of prosthetic heart valves.[14,15] These valves are now in widespread use and there are numerous different designs. Evaluation of prosthetic valve function by catheter methods can be more difficult than with native valves and there is an increased potential for morbidity from the catheter investigation in these patients.

Mechanical valves

These may be of the ball and cage type (e.g. Starr-Edwards) or the tilting metallic disc type (e.g. Bjork-Shilley single leaflet or Carbomedic bileaflet valve). All forms of mechanical valve produce intense echoes from their components and it is often difficult to achieve high resolution imaging of the valve mechanism itself. It is usually possible to assess the movement of the valve cage and valve ring and it is usually possible to see with moderate clarity the movement of the leaflets or ball valve. Abnormal movement of the valve ring can be an important sign of paraprosthetic leak or of valve detachment. This type of abnormality can be further evaluated using Doppler studies and in particular colour flow examination has proved invaluable in the assessment of position and severity of prosthetic valve leaks.

In some cases valve mechanisms become restricted by thrombus or other tissue encroachment and this will lead to a stenotic prosthesis. Reduced movement of the valve components can sometimes be seen and stenosis itself can be calculated using continuous wave Doppler examination as described above. In the evaluation of mechanical prostheses it should be remembered that the intensely echogenic material of the valve will shield the region behind it and so any assessment of flow (particularly regurgitation) will be affected by this and multiple echo windows should be used to ensure a full search for regurgitant jets. In the case of assessing possible prosthetic stenosis it should be remembered that most prostheses have a mild gradient and are essentially equivalent to a mildly stenotic native valve (Fig. 11). It is therefore necessary to understand the range of normality that should be expected with various types of prostheses.

In the case of Starr-Edwards (ball valve) and Bjork Shilley (tilting disc) valves, the major flow through the valve does not

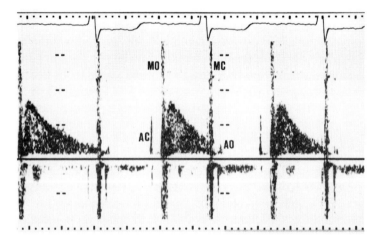

Fig. 11 Apical continuous wave trace from a patient with a normally functioning prosthetic mitral valve. The flow trace shows a typical mildly stenotic pattern. Prominent valve opening (MO) and closing (MC) artefacts are seen. The continuous wave beam has also recorded the aortic opening (AO) and closing (AC) artefacts.

occur centrally and thus a perfectly aligned Doppler beam will not necessarily give a satisfactory recording of transvalvular flow. It will be necessary to adjust the angulation in order to detect the greatest possible jet velocity through the valve; once this is done the calculations regarding pressure gradients can be made.

Biological valves

The majority of biological valves are porcine xenografts but in a minority of cases calf pericardium is used for the construction of the valve leaflets. Human homograft aortic valves are occasionally used. In the former two cases the biological valve leaflets are mounted on a mechanical stent which can be echogenic in the same way that a mechanical prosthesis is echogenic. The leaflets them-selves however, are thin and can often be recorded showing normal movement similar to that observed in a normal aortic valve (Fig. 12). There are normally three prosthetic leaflets in each valve and these open in a similar fashion to the aortic valve so that flow

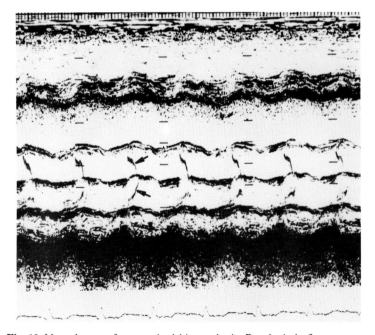

Fig. 12 M-mode trace from a mitral bioprosthesis. Prosthetic leaflet movement (arrowed) is seen within the heavy reflections from the supporting stent.

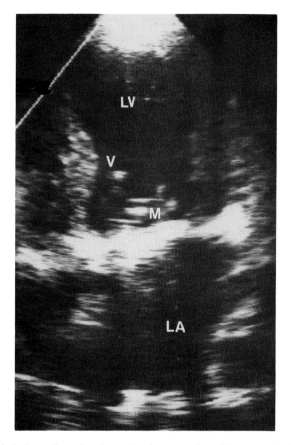

Fig. 13 Apical two dimensional scan showing vegetations (V) on a prosthetic mitral valve (M). The left ventricle (LV) and left atrium (LA) are labelled.

occurs centrally through the valve and normal Doppler alignments can be made.

In all forms of prosthetic valve there is a high risk of infection and the detection of vegetations can be more difficult than with native valves due to the echogenic nature of the material. Nevertheless careful examination will often reveal mobile vegetations in the case of endocarditis (Fig. 13).

SUMMARY

Modern instruments can now give extremely full evaluation of intracardiac valve abnormalities particularly when comprehensive

Doppler facilities including colour flow mapping are available.[16] This situation has a great impact on practice in the catheterisation laboratory. If adequate quality ultrasound studies are carried out it should not be necessary for a patient with cardiac valve disease to reach the catheterisation laboratory without a comprehensive haemodynamic diagnosis. In some cases catheterisation will not be required at all.

Cardiac catheterisation should therefore be used increasingly selectively in patients with cardiac valve disease. The coronary arterial tree cannot be adequately assessed echocardiographically and thus if there is any possibility of coronary disease then arteriography must be performed in pre-operative cases. It must be remembered however, that coronary arteriography alone is a relatively short and straightforward procedure in experienced hands. The addition of catheter evaluation of valve disease can often prolong examinations considerably and it may not be necessary to perform all the usual haemodynamic protocols required in the past.

A patient with severe aortic stenosis, for example, can have the valve gradient calculated, the left ventricle assessed and the mitral valve function evaluated without catheterisation. In this situation the only further information required by the cardiac surgeon will concern the coronary arterial tree. In a young patient it may not be needed at all.

In some cases cardiac catheterisation cannot give such precise information as Doppler studies, particularly when technical problems have occurred during the cardiac catheter. Mitral regurgitation occurring during a run of ventricular ectopics whilst the left ventricular angiogram is being performed can often be hard to assess but this can be simplified with Doppler examination. Mitral valve pressure half time together with mean gradient estimation will often give more precise information about mitral stenosis than the pulmonary wedge pressure.

In spite of this there will be some situations in which confirmatory evidence is required from cardiac catheter. In some circumstances this will be because of a difficult or poor quality echocardiographic examination. The need for catheterisation should thus be evaluated in the light of available echocardiographic information.

Acute valvular pathology is particularly well suited to non-invasive ultrasound examination. Cardiac catheterisation in patients with acute infective endocarditis have a higher than usual morbidity. Acute aortic valve pathology secondary to aortic root pathology is associated with higher than average risk in the catheterisation laboratory where in some cases prosthetic valve disruption is difficult to examine. In these situations direct operative intervention will often follow the ultrasound examination. The recent introduction of trans-oesophageal ultrasound probes has widened the scope for cardiac ultrasound investigation. Although the technique is to a certain extent 'invasive', there will frequently be situations when the addition of information by this method will be preferable to cardiac catheterisation.

Full cardiac valve evaluation is therefore a matter of careful assessment of the management requirements for any individual patient and investigations must be selected appropriately. There is no advantage in adding the modern technology of cardiac ultrasound scanning to the investigation protocols of valve patients if there is no actual or potential benefit by the reduction in the amount of invasive investigation that is carried out on the patients.

REFERENCES

1 Griffiths JM, Henry WL. A sector scanner for real time two dimensional echocardiography. Circulation 1974; 49: 1147–1150
2 Griffiths JM, Henry WL. An ultrasound system for combined imaging and Doppler flow measurement in man. Circulation 1978; 57: 925–928
3 Hatle L, Angelsen B. Doppler ultrasound in cardiology. New York: Lea and Febiger, 1985
4 Holen J, Aaslid R, Landmark K, Simonsen S. Determination of pressure gradient in mitral stenosis with a noninvasive ultrasound Doppler technique. Acta Med Scand 1976; 199: 455–457
5 Hatle L, Angelsen B, Tromsdal A. Noninvasive assessment of atrioventricular pressure half-time by Doppler ultrasound. Circulation 1979; 60: 1096–1102
6 Nichol PM, Boughner DR, Persaud JA. Non-invasive assessment of mitral insufficiency by transcutaneous Doppler ultrasound. Circulation 1976; 54: 656–660
7 Helmke F, Nanda NC, Hsuing MC et al. Color Doppler assessment of mitral regurgitation with orthogonal planes. Circulation 1987; 75: 175–179
8 Simpson IA, Houston AB, Sheldon CD, Hutton I, Lawne TDV. Clinical value of Doppler Echocardiography in the assessment of adults with aortic stenosis. Br Heart J 1984; 53: 636–642
9 Pridie RB, Benham R, Oakley CM. Echocardiography of the mitral valve in aortic valve disease. Br Heart J 1971; 33: 296–300
10 Hoffman A, Pfisterer M, Stulz P, Schmitt HE, Burkart F, Burkhardt D. Noninvasive grading of aortic regurgitation by Doppler ultrasonography. Br Heart J 1986; 55: 283–286
11 Masuyama T, Kodama K, Kitabatake A et al. Noninvasive evaluation of aortic regurgitation by continuous wave Doppler echocardiography. Circulation 1986; 73: 460–463
12 Touche T, Prasquier R, Nitenberg A, de Zuttere D, Gourgon R. Assessment and follow up of patients with aortic regurgitation by an updated echocardiog-

raphic measurement of the regurgitant fraction in the aortic arch. Circulation 1985; 72: 819–824

13 Waggoner AD, Quinones MA, Young JB et al. Pulsed Doppler echocardiographic detection of right-sided valve regurgitation. Am J Cardiol 1981; 472: 79–83

14 Veyrat C, Witchitz S, Lessana A, Ameur A, Abitbol G, Kalmanson D. Valvar prosthetic dysfunction: localisation and evaluation of the dysfunction using the Doppler technique. Br Heart J 1985; 54: 273–278

15 Wilkins GT, Gillam LD, Kritzer GL, Levine RA, Palacios IF, Weyman AE. Validation of continuous wave Doppler echocardiographic measurements of mitral and tricuspid prosthetic valve gradients: a simultaneous Doppler-catheter study. Circulation 1986; 74: 786–790

16 Wilde P. Doppler Echocardiography: an illustrated clinical guide. Edinburgh: Churchill Livingstone, 1989

British Medical Bulletin (1989) Vol. 45, No. 4, pp. 1036–1060
© The British Council 1989

Cross-sectional echocardiography

M L Rigby
A N Redington
Brompton Hospital, London, UK

Cross-sectional echocardiography has become an essential part of the investigation of infants and children with heart disease. Frequently, it provides a precise diagnosis. In many instances, particularly in neonates and infants, surgery can be undertaken without the need to proceed to cardiac catheterisation.[1,2] Although cross-sectional echocardiography provides little information about pulmonary or systemic vascular resistance and flow, considerable information about the latter can be established by Doppler.[3] Echocardiography is essentially the representation of cardiac morphology in life. This technique can, therefore, readily be used in sequential segmental analysis of all patients.

SEQUENTIAL SEGMENTAL ANALYSIS

The ideal terminology for complex congenital heart disease allows an easy, accurate and unambiguous description of all known hearts. It is now generally accepted that sequential segmental analysis[4,5] fulfils these criteria, although there is still some disagreement as to how this method should be utilized and which terms should be used for the categorization of chamber relationships and interconnexions of the cardiac segments.[6] A commonly accepted scheme for the classification of complex congenital cardiac anomalies is shown in Table 1.[7] In the clinical context, bronchial anatomy determined by penetrated radiographs of the chest is a useful guide to the determination of atrial arrangement[8] but cross-sectional echocardiographic assessment of the relationships of the abdominal great vessels at level T10 permits the differentiation of the four types of atrial situs (usual, mirror-image, left or right isomerism).[9]

0007–1420/89/0045–1036/$10.00

Table 1

Atrial arrangement (Situs)
  Usual (solitus)
  Mirror-image (inversus)
  Right isomerism
  Left isomerism
Type of atrioventricular connexion
  Biventricular: Concordant
                Discordant
                Ambiguous (with atrial isomerism)
  Univentricular: Double inlet   ] Dominant LV
                Absent right connexion] Dominant RV
                Absent left connexion] Solitary indeterminate ventricle
Mode of atrioventricular connexion
  Two atrioventricular valves:
                  Normal   (one or both valves)
                  Imperforate (one valve)
                  Stenotic   (one or both valves)
                  Prolapsing (one or both valves)
                  Straddling (one or both valves)
                  Overriding (one or both valves)
  Common valve:
                  Overriding
                  Straddling
                  Stenotic
                  Prolapsing
  Solitary valve (with absent right or left connexion):
                  Normal
                  Overriding
                  Straddling
                  Prolapsing
Type of ventriculo-arterial connexion
  Concordant
  Discordant
  Double outlet ventricle (left, right or indeterminate)
  Single outlet: Pulmonary atresia
               Aortic atresia
               Common arterial trunk
               Solitary arterial trunk
Mode of ventriculo-arterial connexion
  Imperforate valve
  Stenotic valve
  Prolapsing valve

DETERMINATION OF ATRIAL ARRANGEMENT

By recording horizontal abdominal echocardiographic sections at the level of the 10th or 11th thoracic vertebra, the relationship of the abdominal great vessels can be used to infer thoracic and, therefore, atrial arrangement. The aorta can usually be recognized by its pulsations which are synchronous with the movement of the cardiac apex. The inferior caval vein expands with inspiration. When horizontal sections through the abdomen show symmetrical positions of the aorta and inferior caval vein anterior to the spine, lateralized atrial arrangement can be assumed. The morphologically right atrium is then on the side of the inferior caval vein. Thus for usual atrial arrangement (solitus) the aorta is to the left and the inferior caval vein to the right. But in the presence of mirror image arrangement of the atria (inversus) the aorta will be to the right while the inferior caval vein is to the left (Fig. 1). These relationships can be confirmed by sagittal echocardiographic sections which will also demonstrate the inferior caval vein draining directly to the morphological right atrium (Fig. 2).

When there is right atrial isomerism, the aorta and inferior caval vein are frequently found to the same side of the spine with the vein slightly anterior but still draining directly to one of the morphologically right atria (Fig. 3). A midline aorta in the presence of interruption of the inferior caval vein and continuation via a large lateral and posterior azygous vein is characteristic of left isomerism (Fig. 4). Thus in atrial isomerism symmetrical arrangement of the abdominal great vessels does not occur. In right isomerism there is an inferior caval vein anterior to the aorta, whereas in left isomerism there is a large azygous vein posterior to the aorta. This latter pattern may occasionally be found with lateralized atria. Therefore, attention must also be given to the connection of the hepatic veins. When there is lateralized arrangement or right isomerism, some or all of the hepatic veins drain to

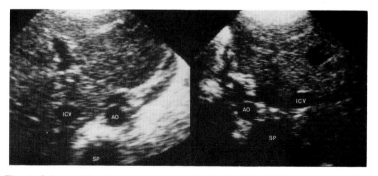

Fig. 1 Subcostal horizontal sections at the level of the 12th thoracic vertebra showing a right-sided inferior caval vein (ICV) and left-sided aorta (AO) and their relationship to the spine (SP) in usual atrial arrangement (solitus). The right hand figure shows a right-sided aorta and left-sided inferior caval vein in mirror image arrangement (situs inversus)

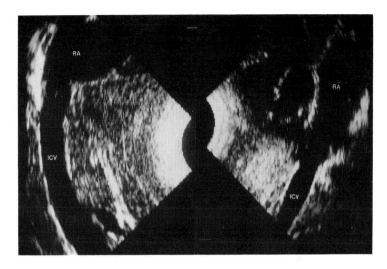

Fig. 2 Subcostal parasagittal sections showing a right-sided inferior caval vein (ICV) draining to a right-sided morphologically right atrium (RA) in usual atrial arrangement (solitus). The right hand figure shows a left-sided inferior caval vein draining to a left-sided morphologically right atrium in mirror image atrial arrangement (inversus)

the inferior caval vein. In the presence of left atrial isomerism, the hepatic veins drain directly to the atria. This pattern also permits the detection of left isomerism when the inferior caval vein is not interrupted. The course of the hepatic veins can be traced using the subcostal four chamber scans.

TYPE OF ATRIOVENTRICULAR CONNEXION

When the atrial arrangement has been determined, the echocardiographic analysis proceeds with determination of the atrioventricular connexion. Here there are two major options, each with its own set of subcategories. Firstly, each atrium may connect to a separate ventricle, irrespective of the nature of the valves guarding the junction. This is termed a biventricular atrioventricular connexion. A concordant connexion exists when the morphologically right atrium is connected to the morphologically right ventricle and the morphologically left atrium is connected to the morphologically left ventricle. The atrioventricular connexion is discordant when the right atrium is connected to the morphologically left ventricle and the left atrium to the morphologically right ventricle.

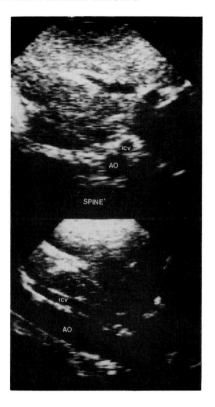

Fig. 3 Horizontal and parasagittal sections in right isomerism showing the aorta (AO) and anterior inferior caval vein (ICV) to the same side of the spine

For a biventricular atrioventricular connexion with lateralized atrial chambers concordant or discordant connexions are the only options.

When there is atrial isomerism with each atrium connecting to a separate ventricle, then the connexion cannot be either concordant or discordant because one of the atria must connect to a morphologically inappropriate ventricle. This arrangement is termed an ambiguous atrioventricular connexion. Having determined the atrioventricular connexion it is then necessary to describe the position of the right ventricle relative to the left.

The echocardiographic determination of the type of atrioventricular connexion is determined from parasternal, apical and subcostal four chamber sections. The mitral valve (which forms an integral part of the morphologically left ventricle) has chordal

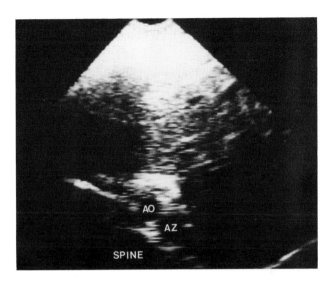

Fig. 4 Subcostal horizontal sections demonstrating an anterior aorta (AO) and posterior azygous vein (AZ) in left atrial isomerism

attachments to two discrete left ventricular papillary muscles and chordae do not insert into the septum. In contrast the tricuspid valve has chordal attachments to the right ventricular aspect of the septum (Fig. 5). In most hearts with biventricular atrioventricular connexion, the demonstration of the presence or absence of the chordal attachments to the septum allows the morphology of the atrioventricular valves, and hence the ventricles to be determined. Another technique to assess the morphology of the atrioventricular valves is to examine the basal attachment of their septal leaflets. The septal leaflet of the tricuspid valve is attached slightly nearer to the apex of the heart than is the corresponding leaflet of the mitral valve. Providing that there is not a perimembranous inlet ventricular septal defect, this offsetting of the atrioventricular valves enables the mitral and tricuspid valves to be distinguished (Fig. 6). There are still other but less reliable methods of identifying ventricular morphology by echocardiography. The left ventricle is typified by its smooth trabecular pattern with two paired papillary muscles, while the right ventricle is coarsely trabeculated with unequal papillary muscles and has the moderator band at its apex. Short axis sections may identify a trileaflet tricuspid valve in contrast to a bileaflet mitral valve. Thus knowing atrial arrangement and ventricular morphology the various types of biventricu-

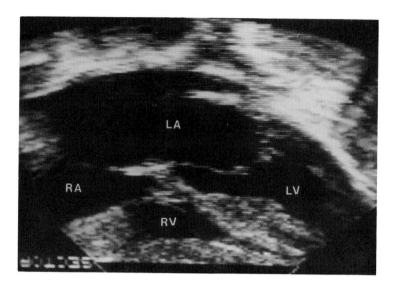

Fig. 5 Subcostal four chamber section showing the left atrium (LA) connected to the left ventricle (LV) with no chordal insertions to the ventricular septum. In contrast the right atrium (RA) connects to the right ventricle (RV) through the tricuspid valve which does have chordal insertions to the ventricular septum

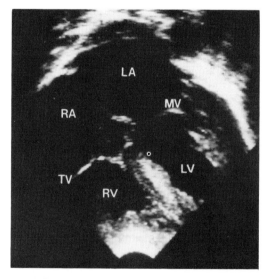

Fig. 6 Parasternal four chamber section showing the usual offsetting of the tricuspid valve (TV) and mitral valve (MV). Thus the muscular and membranous parts of the atrioventricular septum can be seen separating the right atrium (RA) from left ventricle (LV). LA = left atrium; RV = right ventricle

lar atrioventricular connexion can be described along with the relationship of the ventricles.

When describing the atrioventricular connexion a second set of options is available for the atrial chambers to connect with the ventricular mass. A univentricular atrioventricular connexion exists when the atrial chambers connect to only one ventricle.[10] The possible connexions are double inlet ventricle, absence of the right sided atrioventricular connexion or absence of the left sided connexion. A univentricular connexion is most readily demonstrated by four chamber echocardiographic sections. For hearts with absent right connexion, the majority of which are examples of classical tricuspid atresia, there is no potential connexion between the floor of the right sided atrium and the ventricular mass (Fig. 7). Atrioventricular sulcus tissue interposes between them. Similarly, when there is absence of the left atrioventricular connexion sulcus tissue can be demonstrated between the left sided atrium and the ventricular mass (Fig. 8). When both atria are shown to connect directly to one ventricle, either through separate right and left atrioventricular valves or (less frequently) through a common valve, the atrioventricular connexion is de-

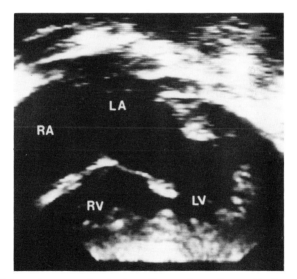

Fig. 7 Subcostal cross-sectional echocardiogram from a heart with absence of the right atrioventricular connexion. Sulcus tissue interposes between the floor of the right atrium (RA) and the ventricular mass. LA = left atrium; LV = left ventricle; RV = right ventricle

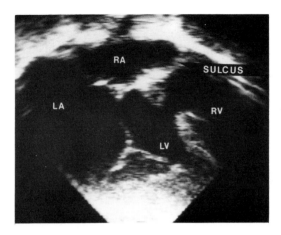

Fig. 8 Parasternal four chamber section from a heart with absence of the left atrioventricular connexion showing sulcus tissue interposing between the floor of the right atrium (RA) and the ventricular mass. The morphologically left atrium (LA) connects to the left ventricle (LV) through the solitary right atrioventricular valve. An interventricular communication can be seen connecting the left ventricle to the right ventricle (RV).

scribed as double inlet (Figs. 9, 10). The majority of these hearts possess a second rudimentary ventricle. This can usually be demonstrated to the right or left of the dominant ventricle by apical, parasternal and subcostal four chamber sections. A rudimentary right ventricle found in hearts with univentricular connexion to a left ventricle will be seen anterosuperiorly in parasternal long and short axis and in subcostal views (Fig. 11). When there is a univentricular atrioventricular connexion to a dominant right ventricle, similar sections will demonstrate a postero-inferior rudimentary left ventricle (Fig. 12). It is the identification of the position of the rudimentary ventricle which is the most reliable echocardiographic guide to the morphology of the dominant ventricle.[11] Occasionally, there is no second rudimentary ventricle identified. It may then be assumed that the atria are connected to a solitary and indeterminate ventricle, although rarely rudimentary ventricles may be present but too small to be visualized by echocardiography.

It is important to emphasize that the type of univentricular atrioventricular connexion is independent both of atrial arrangement and ventricular morphology. Thus, for example, although in the majority of hearts with usual atrial arrangement an absence of the right atrioventricular connexion the morphologically left

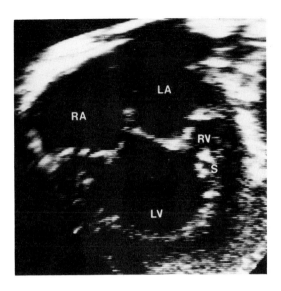

Fig. 9 Subcostal cross-sectional echocardiographic section from a heart with usual atrial arrangement and double inlet left ventricle so that both the right atrium (RA) and left atrium (LA) connect to a morphologically left ventricle (LV). There is a small and rudimentary right ventricle (RV) and the ventricular septum (S) can be identified

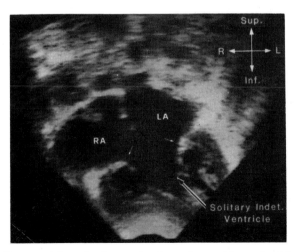

Fig. 10 Parasternal four chamber section from a heart with usual atrial arrangement in which the atria connect to a solitary and indeterminate ventricle through a common atrioventricular valve (arrow). RA = right atrium; LA = left atrium

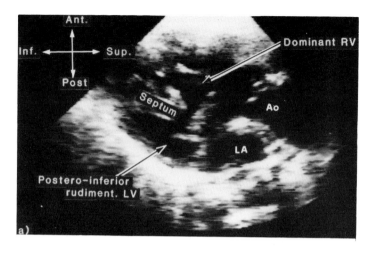

Fig. 11 Parasternal long axis section from a heart with univentricular atrioventricular connexion to a dominant right ventricle in which there is a postero-inferior rudimentary left ventricle. LA = left atrium; AO = aorta

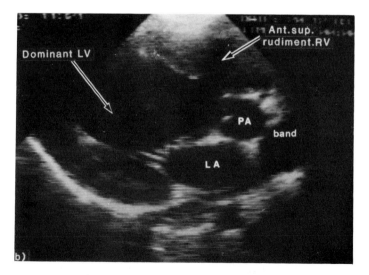

Fig. 12 Parasternal long axis section from a heart with univentricular atrioventricular connexion to a dominant left ventricle in which there is an anterior and superior rudimentary right ventricle. There is a band on the pulmonary artery (PA). LA = left atrium

atrium connects to the morphologically left ventricle, the left atrium may connect to a dominant right ventricle or an indeterminate ventricle.

MODE OF ATRIOVENTRICULAR CONNEXION

Having determined the type of atrioventricular connexion the next step in sequential segmental analysis is to describe the mode of connexion. Whereas the term 'type' of connexion is used to describe the way that the atria connect to the ventricles, the term 'mode' of connexion describes the morphology of the valves which guard the atrioventricular junction. Cross-sectional echocardiography is particularly suited to the demonstration of abnormalities of the atrioventricular valves, usually by means of four chamber sections. An imperforate valve is one which allows potential anatomical continuity between an atrium and a ventricle. Characteristically it is seen to 'balloon' into the ventricle during atrial systole. In a few cases hypoplastic tensor apparatus may be identified attached to the ventricular aspect of the membrane. An atrioventricular valve may also override and/or straddle the ventricular septum and in these circumstances there is almost always malalignment between the atrial and the ventricular septal structures so that a ventricular septal defect is present. In order to describe a valve as straddling, tensor apparatus must be seen to arise from both ventricles. Cross-sectional echocardiography readily allows the distinction of biventricular and univentricular atrioventricular connexions in hearts with an overriding valve. When there are two atrioventricular valves, it is the 50% rule which is envoked to make the distinction. In the presence of a common valve, then less than 75% of the valve annulus should be connected to one ventricle in order to describe the connexion as biventricular. The various modes of connexion are listed in Table 1 and includes stenotic and prolapsing valves.

TYPE OF VENTRICULO-ARTERIAL CONNEXION

Having determined atrial arrangement, the type of atrioventricular connexion and the mode of connexion, the next step in the diagnostic pathway is the description of the type of ventriculoarterial connexion. It is necessary first to identify ventricular morphology by the methods already described. A concordant connexion is described when the morphologically right ventricle gives rise to the pulmonary trunk and the morphologically left ventricle to the aorta. A discordant ventriculo-arterial connexion describes a situation where the aorta arises from the morphologically right ventricle and the pulmonary trunk from the morphologically left ventricle (Fig. 13). Double outlet exists when both of the great arteries arise from the same ventricle (Fig. 14) which may be a morphologically right ventricle, a morphologically left ventricle or a solitary indeterminate ventricle. Single outlet heart

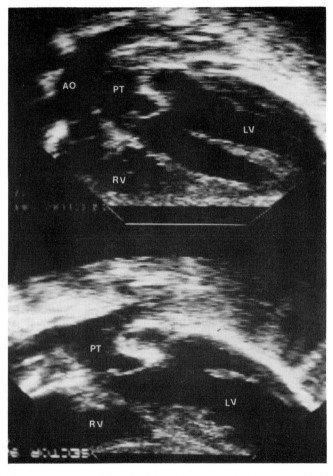

Fig. 13 Subcostal long axis section from a heart with complete transposition of the great arteries showing the pulmonary trunk (PT) connected to the morphologically left ventricle (LV) and the aorta (AO) arising from the morphologically right ventricle (RV)

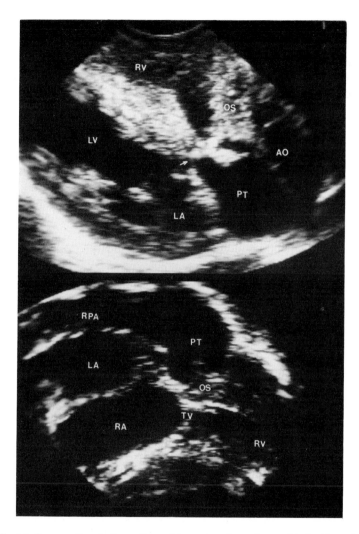

Fig. 14 Cross-sectional echocardiographic sections from a heart with double outlet right ventricle. The upper figure shows both the aorta (AO) and pulmonary trunk (PT) arising from the morphologically right ventricle (RV). There is a huge outlet septum (OS) causing subaortic stenosis. The outlet from the left ventricle (LV) is a restrictive ventricular septal defect (arrow). LA = left atrium. The lower figure is a subcostal section which demonstrates the outlet septum (OS), the pulmonary trunk (PT) and the right pulmonary artery (RPA). Also identifiable are the left atrium (LA), right atrium (RA) and tricuspid valve (TV)

describes a situation where only one arterial trunk is in connexion with the ventricular mass. The most important examples are a common arterial trunk (Fig. 15), and pulmonary atresia or aortic atresia when it is impossible to trace any potential ventricular connexion of the atretic trunk. A solitary arterial trunk exists when there are no central intrapericardial pulmonary arteries, so that it is impossible to determine if the solitary trunk is a common trunk or an aorta.

In order to determine the type of ventriculo-arterial connexion by cross-sectional echocardiography, the nature of the arterial trunk or trunks must be determined. The pulmonary trunk is recognized by demonstrating its bifurcation into right and left branches. The aorta is identified by visualizing its ascending portion and arch along with its branches. A common arterial trunk is a single great artery which gives rise directly in its ascending part to coronary and pulmonary arteries and continues as the ascending aorta. In practice it is relatively easy in infants to demonstrate the origin of the great arteries by recording subcostal outlet sections. From this position the bifurcation of the pulmonary trunk can be identified together with the ascending aorta and

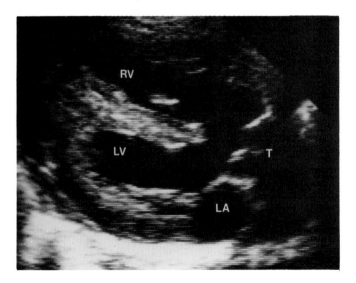

Fig. 15 Parasternal long axis section from a heart with a common arterial trunk. The solitary common arterial trunk (T) overrides the ventricular septum so that it arises equally from the morphologically right ventricle (RV) and left ventricle (LA). LA = left atrium

proximal arch. Thus, ventriculo-arterial concordance or ventriculo-arterial discordance (Fig. 13) can usually be established using this approach. Although in older children the great arteries are not so readily demonstrated in this fashion, the ventriculo-arterial connexion can usually be established by combining subcostal, parasternal and apical long axis sections of the ventricles and great arteries, together with suprasternal or high parasternal long axis sections of the aorta and pulmonary arteries. When an abnormal ventriculo-arterial connexion is associated with a perimembranous ventricular septal defect, subcostal sections may give the erroneous impression of double outlet ventricle when the ventriculo-arterial connexion is really concordant or discordant. For this reason the diagnosis of abnormalities of ventriculo-arterial connexion associated with a ventricular septal defect must be established by parasternal long axis sections which show both ventricles, the ventricular septum and the origin of both great arteries. When there is an overriding arterial trunk the 50% rule is used to determine its origin either from the left or right ventricle.

MODE OF VENTRICULO-ARTERIAL CONNEXION

In similar fashion to the mode of atrioventricular connexion, the term 'mode of ventriculo-arterial connexion' describes the morphology of the semilunar valves which guard the ventriculo-arterial junction. However, at the ventriculo-arterial junction the modes of connexion are much more limited. When there are two arterial valves, one of them may be imperforate and either or both may override the ventricular septum. An imperforate valve is the common form of arterial valve atresia but in the circumstances the ventriculo-arterial connexion should still be concordant, discordant or double outlet. Other abnormalities of modes of connexion include stenotic or prolapsing semilunar valves.

THE SUBARTERIAL INFUNDIBULUM

Having established the ventriculo-arterial connexion the infundibular morphology must then be described. Several possibilities exist. There may be bilateral infundibula, bilaterally deficient infundibula, a subaortic infundibulum or finally a subpulmonary infundibulum. The description of these depends upon subcostal outlet sections and parasternal long axis sections.

The infundibular septum is that part of the ventricular septum which divides the outlets of the morphologically right and left ventricles. Insignificant when the ventricular septum is intact, it is easily demonstrated by cross-sectional echocardiography when it is separate from the rest of the septum. Its morphology is fundamental to the understanding of outflow tract obstruction and abnormalities of ventriculo-arterial connexion, both in the setting of biventricular and univentricular atrioventricular connexion. Anterior or posterior deviation of the outlet septum produces a malalignment ventricular septal defect and has the potential to cause subarterial obstruction (Fig. 16).

ASSOCIATED LESIONS

Having described the atrial arrangement and the type and mode of atrioventricular and ventriculo-arterial connexions, the associated lesions must then be categorized. In the majority of abnormal hearts the chamber connexions and relationships are normal. There are only the 'associated lesion(s)' to be described. These are generally listed in logical sequence beginning with abnormalities of systemic or pulmonary venous drainage and progressing through atrial anomalies, atrioventricular septal defects, abnormalities of the atrioventricular valves, ventricular anomalies and abnormalities of the great arteries and their branches. Functional abnormalities of the ventricles should also be described.

ECHOCARDIOGRAPHY IN THE NEONATE AND INFANT

The vast majority of congenital heart anomalies are now detected during the first year of life.

It has been outlined already how cross-sectional echocardiography may be used in the sequential segmental analysis in hearts with a wide variety of differing morphology. This is especially true in neonates and infants in whom a precise diagnosis can frequently be made based upon physical examination, inspection of the electrocardiogram and chest radiograph, and cross-sectional echocardiography. Before the advent of modern echocardiography, cardiac catheterisation and angiography were the standard methods of diagnosis in symptomatic neonates and infants; they could be considered the final arbiter. Today in many instances the final arbiter in morphological diagnosis is cross-sectional echocardiog-

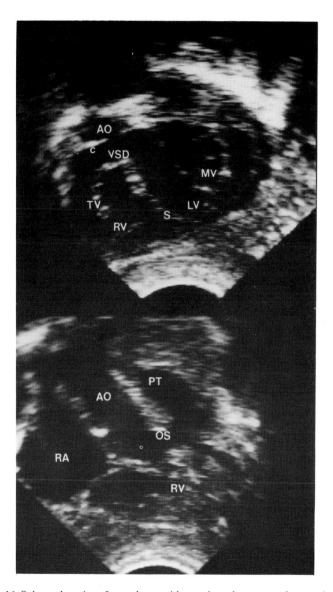

Fig. 16 Subcostal sections from a heart with a perimembranous outlet ventricular septal defect. The upper figure shows the perimembranous ventricular septal defect with its posterior margin the central fibrous body (C). MV = mitral valve; LV = left ventricle; S = ventricular septum; RV = right ventricle; TV = tricuspid valve. The lower figure is a subcostal right oblique section which demonstrates both the aorta (AO) and pulmonary trunk (PT) and the outlet septum (OS). The outlet septum is clearly defined because it is malaligned from the rest of the ventricular septum. RA = right atrium; RV = right ventricle

raphy, while cardiac catheterisation provides more precise information about flows and resistances when it is required.

Bearing in mind, therefore, the extensive capabilities of echocardiography, several important questions must be answered. Firstly, what are its limitations? Secondly, under which circumstances may cardiac catheterisation be avoided? And, thirdly, what contribution does Doppler echocardiography provide in the diagnosis of heart disease in the neonate and infant.

LIMITATIONS OF ECHOCARDIOGRAPHY

It is self evident that the limitations of echocardiography are, in part, related to the experience and skill of the operator and the capabilities of the equipment. Exactly the same is true of cardiac catheterisation and angiography. For the purpose, therefore, of this discussion it must be presumed that the personnel are experienced and the equipment is the best that is currently available. No physician or surgeon would consider an item of diagnostic information in isolation. It must be assumed, therefore, that clinical information and at least a high quality chest X-ray and electrocardiogram are available for study.

Having then set the conditions, what are the general limitations of echocardiography in the diagnosis of neonates and infants? It fails to permit the diagnosis of regurgitation of the atrioventricular valves and may be unreliable in determining the severity of atrioventricular valve stenosis and ventricular outflow tract obstruction. The detection of small muscular ventricular septal defects may be impossible. And echocardiography is less suitable than angiography for the demonstration of the aorta and distal pulmonary arteries. Also, it does not provide direct information about pulmonary and systemic blood flow or pulmonary vascular resistance. This latter information, however, may not be required. Doppler echocardiography is a valuable adjunct to standard echocardiography providing both qualitative and quantitative information.

Let us consider, for example, a four month old infant with a complete atrioventricular septal defect (AV canal defect) presenting with failure to thrive and congestive heart failure. The chest radiography shows cardiac enlargement with markedly increased pulmonary vascular markings. In such a case the measurement of pulmonary blood flow is quite irrelevant to the management of the patient. There are three major management options. Firstly, complete correction, secondly, banding of the pulmonary artery and, thirdly, medical management alone when there is associated Down's syndrome.[12-14] If banding of the pulmonary artery is the preferred treatment then a contra-indication to this procedure might be a large intracardiac shunt from left ventricle to right atrium. This might be evident on cardiac catheterisation and angiography or could, perhaps, be detected by Doppler; although there is no evidence to show that either technique can successfully select those few patients who are unsuitable for this palliative procedure. In this case, therefore, clinical assessment and echocardiography probably provide sufficient data to allow pulmonary artery banding to be performed with minimal risk to the patient. Alternatively, it may be the policy of the unit to advise corrective surgery for most infants with atrioventricular canal defects. In a minority of cases there will be an additional muscular ventricular septal defect or multiple defects. It is well recognized that cross-sectional echocardiography may fail to demonstrate these additional defects. Doppler echocardiography is also unreliable. Cardiac catheterisation prior to corrective surgery can, therefore, be justified in the best interests of the patient. It is our policy, however, to proceed to cardiac catheterisation only if a high quality echocardiogram is not obtained although in practice infants with atrioventricular septal defects are extremely 'echogenic' and angiography is frequently not required.

In marked contrast to the case that has been presented an older infant with the same lesion but not demonstrating failure to thrive, heart failure and marked pulmonary plethora on the chest radiograph provides a different problem. The absence of heart failure may result from the presence of right ventricular outflow tract obstruction, a raised pulmonary vascular resistance or a limiting interventricular component. If cross-sectional echocardiography fails to demonstrate right ventricular outflow tract obstruction or a limiting ventricular septal defect, cardiac catheterisation to measure pulmonary vascular resistance is mandatory if corrective surgery or pulmonary artery banding is being considered. This is because a pulmonary vascular resistance of more than 6 units with the child breathing 100% oxygen is associated with a high operative mortality and progressive pulmonary vascular disease even when surgery is successful.

PALLIATIVE SURGERY WITHOUT PRIOR CARDIAC CATHETERISATION

The two major palliative surgical procedures carried out in symptomatic infants with congenital heart disease are banding of the pulmonary trunk[15] or a systemic artery to pulmonary artery shunt (usually a modified Blalock-Taussig anastomosis).[16]

Banding of the pulmonary artery is performed in infants with unrestricted pulmonary blood flow, often in the setting of more complex congenital heart disease such as hearts with univentricular atrioventricular connexion, congenitally corrected transposition and ventricular septal defect, and multiple ventricular septal defects. In some centres this procedure may also be used for the management of isolated ventricular septal defect, atrioventricular septal defect with common orifice, complete transposition with ventricular septal defect and double outlet right ventricle. By restricting pulmonary blood flow it is frequently an effective treatment for congestive heart failure and failure to thrive. And it carries the important advantage of preventing the development of pulmonary vascular disease, thus allowing definitive surgery to be performed at a later date. Because cross-sectional echocardiography usually allows a precise diagnosis to be made, banding can frequently be carried out without prior cardiac catheterisation and angiography. Under what circumstances, therefore, should cardiac catheterisation be undertaken? The most important indications for invasive study are an echocardiographic diagnosis incompatible with the clinical findings, an incomplete echocardiographic study or the necessity for balloon atrial septostomy in hearts with tricuspid atresia, complete transposition with ventricular septal defect, absence of the left atrioventricular connexion and some conditions with mitral stenosis and hypoplasia of the left ventricle. Even then, balloon atrial septostomy is frequently carried out under echocardiographic screening on an intensive care unit.[17]

A systemic artery to pulmonary artery shunt procedure may be performed in the neonatal period when there is duct dependent pulmonary blood flow or later when restricted pulmonary blood flow results in significant hypoxia. In the majority of cases a modified Blalock-Taussig shunt is the operation of choice. It is carried out when there is pulmonary atresia or severe subpulmonary stenosis. It is applicable, therefore, to hearts with a variety of abnormalities including some with pulmonary atresia and intact septum or ventricular septal defect, hearts with univentricular atrioventricular connexion, tetralogy of Fallot with severe infundibular stenosis, double outlet right ventricle and transposition of the great arteries with associated pulmonary stenosis or atresia.

The major clinical indication for a shunt procedure during the first year of life is severe hypoxia. In order to recommend palliative surgery on the basis of echocardiography alone, the diagnosis must be entirely compatible with the clinical features, severe subpulmonary stenosis or pulmonary atresia should be evident, confluent pulmonary arteries should be demonstrated and the side of the aortic arch should be known. It is wise to remember that contra-indications to the operation may include the presence of associated obstructed total anomalous pulmonary venous return or pulmonary vein stenosis, the former being found frequently when there is right atrial isomerism.

CORRECTIVE NON-BYPASS SURGERY WITHOUT CARDIAC CATHETERISATION

Ligation of an arterial duct, repair of coarctation of the aorta and closed pulmonary valvotomy in hearts with pulmonary atresia and intact septum where there is an imperforate pulmonary valve can usually be undertaken without cardiac catheterisation. In some cases it may be impossible to demonstrate thoracic coarctation even when the clinical features are typical. It is then important to exclude the rare occurrence of abdominal coarctation. An additional problem may be the infant with coarctation and easily palpable femoral pulses because of a widely patent duct caused by the administration of prostaglandins. As always, if in doubt, perform cardiac catheterisation and angiography.

CORRECTIVE BYPASS SURGERY WITHOUT CARDIAC CATHETERISATION

Corrective surgery under cardiopulmonary bypass can be carried out safely in a number of conditions without prior cardiac catheterisation and angiography, providing first class images are obtained by cross-sectional echocardiography. Most importantly, echocardiography may fail to demonstrate additional muscular ventricular septal defects when there is thought to be an isolated ventricular septal defect in, for example, transposition with ventricular septal defect, double outlet right ventricle, atrioventricular septal defect or tetralogy of Fallot. In these conditions, therefore, angiography is usually performed prior to definitive surgery. Currently, however, it is our practice to recommend surgery for infants with large ventricular septal defects or with complete atrioventricular septal defects on the basis of clinical evaluation and cross-sectional echocardiography and Doppler alone. Angiography is particularly useful in the assessment of the size of the pulmonary arteries when there is obstructed pulmonary blood flow (e.g. tetralogy of Fallot) and in the demonstration of coronary artery anomalies.

Angiography is not usually required in hearts with total anomalous pulmonary venous connexion,[18] common arterial trunk, aortopulmonary septal defect (window), interrupted aortic arch, critical aortic stenosis or critical pulmonary stenosis. We usually carry out the arterial switch procedure in neonates with complete transposition on the basis of clinical examination and echocardiography alone.

DOPPLER ECHOCARDIOGRAPHY IN NEONATES AND INFANTS

Doppler provides additional information which cannot always be provided by echocardiography. Most importantly, it identifies regurgitant atrioventricular valves in hearts with both biventricular and univentricular atrioventricular connexion. Under certain circumstances this information may alter the management of the patient. For example, in the newborn with complete transposition the presence of severe tricuspid regurgitation would be considered an indication for an arterial switch procedure. Regurgitation through a common atrioventricular valve in an AV canal defect might be a contra-indication to pulmonary artery banding. Doppler also allows the quantitation of the severity of atrioventricular valve stenosis in infants, although it is usually self evident on cross-sectional echocardiography as well, and the distinction between imperforate and severely stenotic valves. In general Doppler is reliable in the diagnosis of multiple ventricular septal defects when colour flow mapping is employed and excellent in determining the presence of a gradient across a subarterial infundibulum particularly in hearts with abnormalities of ventriculoarterial connexion when duplex scanning with continuous wave Doppler is employed. In theory Doppler should help distinguish an imperforate pulmonary valve in pulmonary atresia with intact septum from critical pulmonary valve stenosis. However, the presence of an arterial duct with a left to right shunt often makes the distinction impossible. Similarly, in the neonate with coarctation and right to left shunting through the arterial duct, Doppler is frequently unreliable in establishing the diagnosis. However, with an isolated arterial duct it is usually diagnostic. Similarly, coarctation is readily diagnosed outside the neonatal period.

In practice, therefore, Doppler does not often radically change the management of the neonate or infant with major congenital heart disease and in general it is not essential to the efficient and safe management of the sick neonate and infant.

REFERENCES

1 Leung MP, Mok CK, Lau KC et al. The role of cross sectional echocardiography and pulsed Doppler ultrasound in the management of neonates in whom congenital heart disease is suspected. Br Heart J 1986; 56: 73–82

2 Gutgesell HP, Huhta JC, Latson LA et al. Accuracy of two-dimensional echocardiography in the diagnosis of congenital heart disease. Am J Cardiol 1985; 55: 514–518

3 Sahn DJ. Real-time 2-dimensional Doppler echocardiographic flow mapping. Circulation 1985; 71: 849–853

4 Van Praagh R, Ongley PA, Swan HJC. Anatomic types of single or common ventricle in man: morphologic and geometric aspects of sixty necropsied cases. Am J Cardiol 1964; 13: 367–386

5 de le Cruz MV, Nadal-Ginard B. Rules for the diagnosis of visceral situs, truncoconal morphologies and ventricular inversions. Am Heart J 1972; 84: 19–32

6 Van Praagh R. Terminology of congenital heart disease: glossary and commentary. Circulation 1977; 56: 139–143

7 Shinebourne EA, Macartney RJ, Anderson RH. Sequential chamber localization — logical approach in diagnosis in congenital heart disease. Br Heart J 1976; 38: 327–340

8 Macartney FJ, Partridge JB, Shinebourne EA et al. Identification of atrial situs. In Anderson RH and Shinebourne EA (eds). Paediatric Cardiology. Churchill Livingstone, Edinburgh, 1978; pp. 16–26

9 Huhta JC, Smallhorn JF, Macartney FJ. Cross-sectional echocardiographic diagnosis of situs. Br Heart J 1982;

10 Anderson RH, Macartney FJ, Tynan MJ et al. Univentricular atrioventricular connection, the single ventricle trap unsprung. Pediatr Cardiol 1985; 4: 273–280

11 Rigby ML, Anderson RH, Gibson D et al. Two-dimensional echocardiographic categorisation of the univentricular heart. Ventricular morphology, type, and mode of atrioventricular connexion. Br Heart J 1981; 46: 603–612

12 Williams WH, Guyton RA, Michalik RE et al. Individualised surgical management of complete atrioventricular canal. J Thorax Cardiovasc Surg 1983; 86: 838–844

13 Mavroudis C, Weinstein G, Turley K, Ebert PA. Surgical management of complete atrioventricular canal. J Thorax Cardiovasc Surg 1982; 83: 670–679

14 Bull C, Rigby ML, Shinebourne EA. Should management of complete atrioventricular canal be influenced by co-existant Down's syndrome. Lancet 1985; I: 1147–1149

15 Muller WH, Dammann JF Jr. The treatment of certain congenital malformations of the heart by creation of pulmonic stenosis to reduce pulmonary hypertension and excessive pulmonary blood flow. Surgery, Gynaecology and Obstetrics 1952; 95: 213–220

16 Blalock A, Taussig HB. The surgical treatment of malformations of the heart in which there is pulmonary stenosis or pulmonary atresia. J Am Med Assoc 1945; 128: 189

17 Allan LD, Leanage R, Wainwright R, Joseph MC, Tynan M. Balloon atrial septostomy under 2-dimensional echocardiographic control. Br Heart J 1982; 47: 41–43

18 Smallhorn JF, Tommasini G, Anderson RH, Macartney FJ. Assessment of atrioventricular septal defects by 2-dimensional echocardiography. Br Heart J 1982; 47: 109–127

British Medical Bulletin (1989) Vol. 45, No. 4, pp. 1061–1075
© The British Council 1989

Assessment of left ventricular structure and function by cross sectional echocardiography

D G Gibson
Brompton Hospital, London, UK

Cross sectional echocardiography can be used to give semiquantitative estimates of ventricular volumes and ejection fraction which are very valuable in detecting the severe abnormalities seen clinically. The technique has also been widely used to study regional abnormalities of wall motion. However, with a frame rate of 30 s^{-1} and lateral resolution of 3–4 mm critical analysis of disturbances of timing is not possible, so the method should be used in conjunction with M-mode and Doppler techniques. In spite of physical limitations, based on the underlying mechanisms of image generation, its advantages of real time application and noninvasive nature, its ability to demonstrate myocardial thickness as well as echo intensity, and its relative cheapness have made cross sectional echocardiography a major tool in documenting abnormalities of left ventricular function occurring in disease.

Clinically occurring left ventricular disease is complex in its genesis. The macroscopic anatomy of the ventricle is nearly always abnormal, with cavity size frequently increased and its shape abnormal. Hypertrophy may be present, either localized or generalized, and the normal highly organized fibre architecture is particularly sensitive to the effects of disease. These disturbances are rarely uniformly distributed, so that incoordinate function is

0007–1420/89/0045–1061/$10.00

common in ventricular disease of all types. Its effect is to submit the myocardial fibres themselves to abnormal loading conditions, thus profoundly altering their function within the heart. It is widely assumed that primary abnormalities of contraction or relaxation also occur in these patients and indeed that they are the main cause of the clinical syndrome of heart failure.[1] Yet, the problem of identifying their presence let alone determining their nature in the structurally abnormal ventricle has proved surprisingly difficult. Even today, the position remains that there is surprisingly little direct evidence for their existence.

There are two main approaches to studying left ventricular disease. Graphical methods, which include phonocardiography, cavity pressure measurements, and external pulsations such as the venous pulse or the apex cardiogram, have proved remarkably sensitive in following abnormalities in the velocity and timing of events and in measuring intervals within the cardiac cycle. They are also very useful in detecting the effects of cardioactive drugs. However, they do not give information about anatomy. To detect abnormal cavity size, shape, and wall thickness, imaging methods are needed. It is with the contribution of cross sectional echocardiography to this problem that the present chapter will be concerned.

LEFT VENTRICULAR CAVITY SIZE

Images of the left ventricular cavity can be obtained by cross sectional echocardiography from parasternal, apical, and subcostal approaches, and can be used to estimate volume in a number of ways. If the cavity is assumed to be ellipsoidal, volume can be calculated in exactly the same way as from a contrast angiogram.[2,3] A rather more sophisticated approach is to use two orthogonal views, usually the apical 2 and 4 chamber cuts. The cavity is outlined in each, and its volume reconstructed using some variant of Simpson's rule. This method avoids assuming any particular geometrical shape.[3-5] An example of its use is given in Figure 1. It can take account of abnormal geometry including reversal of the curvature of cavity outline. Simpsons's rule can also be applied more simply by measuring a series of transverse axes at different levels, usually from parasternal short axis views. The ventricular long axis is obtained from the apical view, and volume reconstructed either as an ellipsoid,[2,3] or by modelling the ventricle as a combination of a cylinder, a truncated cone, and a cone for the

END-DIASTOLIC FRAMES

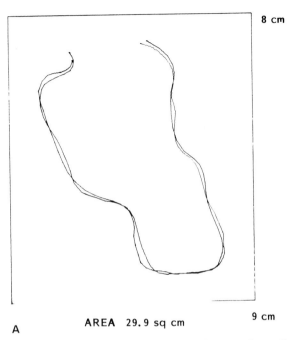

8 cm

AREA 29.9 sq cm

9 cm

A

Fig. 1A Determination of the position of left ventricular cavity outline in two successive beats from end-diastolic frames in a patient with hypertrophic cardiomyopathy, recorded in the apical four chamber view

apex.[4,5] Whatever method is used, estimates of both ventricular volume and also of ejection fraction are consistently lower than those derived from angiography, particularly when values are within the normal range, so that the slope of the regression relation between the two is characteristically between 0.7 and 0.9. For ejection fraction, the standard error of the estimate lies between 5 and 12% (% here meaning ejection fraction units).

All these estimates depend on a set of common manoeuvres. The long axis must be identified and measured in the apical view. The endocardial boundary of the cavity must have been clearly defined, and distinguished from the much higher amplitude echoes arising from the epicardium. In most studies, apical views are used; here the endocardium is defined by backscattered echoes, whose lateral resolution at 3 MHz and a depth of 10–15 cm is only of the order of 3–4 mm. The position of the endocardium is usually taken as

END-DIASTOLE

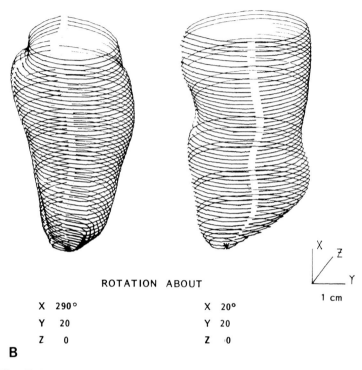

ROTATION ABOUT

X   290°   X   20°

Y   20   Y   20

Z   0   Z   0

B

Fig. 1B Two reconstructions of left ventricular cavity shape from a pair of cavity outlines recorded in apical two and four chamber views. The discontinuity in the circumferential lines represents the position of the original cavity outlines on which the reconstructions are based

corresponding with the 'inside' of these echoes, a questionable assumption. Drop-out is often present, though the missing portion of cavity outline can be interpolated, providing it is not too large.

Although cross sectional echocardiography is widely used to estimate ventricular volume and ejection fraction, problems remain. Estimates are only moderately reproducible with differences of 25–30% between duplicate determinations. This underestimation of volume compared with angiography, is due, in part to foreshortening, since the apex beat, as palpated, does not correspond with the anatomical apex, but with a point approximately one third of the way up the free wall of the ventricle. The limited lateral resolution is another significant factor, particularly when the 'inside' of the endocardial echoes is used to outline the cavity. The image is further corrupted by 'speckle', which is present on all echocardiographic images, giving structures defined by back-scattered echoes their characteristic granular appearance. The exact nature of this speckle pattern is determined only in very small part by the target, but depends almost entirely on the imaging system used. This latter component can, however, be characterized and substantially removed from the image by a process of adaptive filtration.[6] This has the effect of enhancing the endocardial boundary[7] and of increasing the resulting volume estimates by 10–15%. As a result of all these uncertainties, volume estimates based on cross sectional echocardiography should be seen as semiquantitative only, and are useful simply because the range of values seen in disease is so large. The degree of uncertainty associated with them is of the same order as the normal end-systolic volume, so they have no place in assessing the effects of acute interventions on ventricular size or function. An informed guess can agree remarkably well with angiography, particularly if image quality is only moderate.[8]

Cross sectional echocardiography has been much more useful in assessing ventricular cavity shape. Although the normal ventricle is frequently considered to be an ellipsoid of revolution, this is an approximation only. Grant[9] noted that curvature along the inferior wall is reversed, so that it is convex inwards instead of convex outwards as is the rest of the cavity outline. This reversal persists, and indeed is increased during systole, showing that it is not due to any external constraint, such as the diaphragm, but rather that it is a function of the normal myocardial architecture. Its effect is to cause a striking change in cavity shape as cavity volume falls, the convex inferior wall approximating the concave free wall as minor axis falls. This allows a more favourable relation between myocardial shortening or lengthening and volume changes.[10] During ejection, approximately one third of the normal stroke volume is the result of the shape change, while during filling, altering shape towards a more spherical configuration effectively reduces passive chamber stiffness. These changes can be clearly documented by cross sectional echocardiography. Their loss is an early sign of ventricular disease which precedes any fall in ejection fraction in patients with coronary artery disease. More obvious changes in cavity outline are seen when ejection fraction is low. The cavity shape becomes spherical, and does not alter significantly with ejection. The interventricular septum bulges into the right ventricle. Even the earliest cross sectional echo systems were able to detect left ventricular aneurysm formation.[11] Though outward bulging during systole is unusual because aneurysms are fibrotic and thus not distensible at left ventricular pressures, reversal of curvature at the neck is readily apparent. The function of myocardium in the basal region, a primary determinant of survival after operation, can also be assessed.

The pattern of myocardial hypertrophy can also be clearly delineated. Symmetrical hypertrophy, as commonly occurs in hypertension or aortic stenosis, can be distinguished from that predominantly involving the septum in hypertrophic cardiomyopathy. Further patterns have been described. Apical hypertrophic cardiomyopathy is now a well recognised variant, distinguished by the presence of giant negative T waves of the ECG. Less commonly, only the free wall is involved, while a discrete upper septal localization is common in milder forms of both primary and secondary hypertrophy. It has also been possible to document the nature and extent of ventricular remodelling after acute myocardial infarction, a process which may well have a major influence on prognosis, and whose progress may be modified by converting enzyme inhibitors.

REGIONAL WALL MOTION

Regional wall motion can be thought of as consisting of two interrelated components: inward or outward motion of endocardium and thickening or thinning of the underlying myocardium. Although normal ventricular contraction appears symmetrical, clear regional differences in both these components have been demonstrated, affecting their amplitude and timing.[12,13] The significance of these regional differences is still not clear, but they are probably related to optimizing mechanical efficiency and the rate of fluid transfer into and out of the heart. They become impaired with even mild ventricular disease, and their loss may be useful evidence of it. As the disease becomes more severe, so new abnormalities of wall motion develop, affecting both amplitude and timing. Their presence can often be recognized subjectively, and a series of studies have compared cross sectional echo with contrast[14-16] or nuclear[3] angiography in localizing them. Values of 65 to 90% agreement between the two have been reported. In acute myocardial infarction, regional wall motion disturbances usually correspond with the position of Q waves on the ECG[17,18] although in an appreciable number of cases, additional areas of the ventricle are also involved. Their incidence is further increased with exercise, and the reliability with which they can be detected improved by storing end-diastolic and end-systolic images in memory and comparing them directly. It seems, therefore, that such subjective comparison is a useful means of detecting regional disturbances of wall motion, provided that the disturbance is severe and localized as occurs in acute or chronic coronary artery disease. However, it gives little information about their nature.

It would thus seem preferable to use more objective criteria to study wall motion. A series of approaches have been investigated. The simplest is to outline the cavity at end-systole and diastole, and to assess movement between the two. Moynihan et al.[19] describe a method based on the apical 4 chamber and parasternal minor axis views. The endocardial outline is traced with a light pen. Intracardiac landmarks are established on the end-diastolic image; on the minor axis view the midpoint of the left side of the septum, and on the four chamber view the line from the midpoint of the mitral valve to the apex. A second axis is constructed perpendicular to the mid-point of each. Two methods have been used to construct the corresponding axes at end-systole: either the end-diastolic frame of reference was used ('fixed axes') or it was established anew ('floating axes'). Movement can be quantified in terms of shortening of radii or of reduction in the area of each quadrant. Area changes have proved more satisfactory, since the percentage change was greater in comparison with random variation. In normal subjects, the floating axis system gave a more symmetrical pattern of wall motion.

Disturbances in the timing of wall motion are particularly common, particularly in the presence of reversible ischaemia rather than scarring. Extracting such information from cross sectional echocardiographic images has so far proved difficult. Garrison et al.[20] described a method based on parasternal minor axis frames. Endo and epicardial surfaces are first identified manually by superimposing a set of 16 equally spaced points around them, and joined by a 128 point curve. Separate centroids are defined for endo- and epicardium. This process is repeated for each frame of the beat to be studied, and plots are made of endocardial position and wall thickness. More recently, automatic boundary recognition methods have been used.[21,22] Yet another approach has been to consider the information on a two dimensional display as a set of M-mode echocardiograms successively ordered in space rather than a set of cavity outlines ordered in time.[23,24] The multiple M-mode method can readily be implemented, and displays generated giving some idea of the complexity of wall motion in disease (Fig. 2). All these methods have been limited in practice by moderate image quality and by the tedious nature of the analysis when performed manually. This is unfortunate, because there are many circumstances when the information might be of great practical value, such as early after myocardial infarction to assess the progress of thrombolysis,[25] or to monitor treatment of operative or postoperative changes in left ventricular

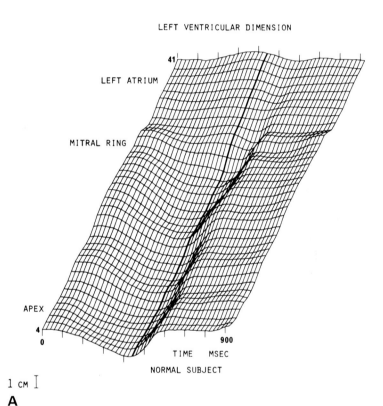

LEFT VENTRICULAR DIMENSION

LEFT ATRIUM

MITRAL RING

APEX

1 CM

TIME   MSEC

NORMAL SUBJECT

A

Fig. 2A Multiple M-mode approach. Horizontal lines represent plots of transverse dimension from the apex of the left ventricle to the upper part of the left atrium. Note the synchronous pattern of change over the left ventricular cavity, with mild delay in dimension increase occurring towards the base of the heart during filling. Vertical lines (isochrones) join events occurring simultaneously on each dimension plot. The accentuated isochrone represents the timing of mitral valve opening

LEFT VENTRICULAR DIMENSION

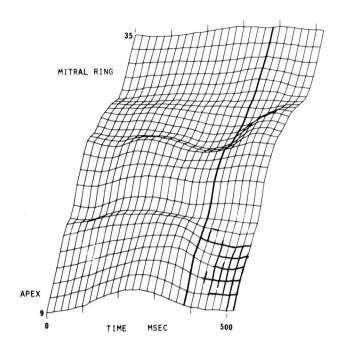

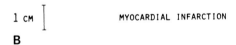

Fig. 2B Multiple M-mode plot from a patient with cardiogenic shock. Note that the normal synchronous pattern of dimension change has been lost, with paradoxical expansion in the mid portion of the cavity

function. It may well be that the much higher quality of left ventricular images obtained by the oesophageal approach may make these methods more practicable.

TISSUE CHARACTERIZATION

Tissue characterization uses echocardiography to gain information about the target echoes beyond simply its position and motion. The technique depends on identifying aspects of the returning echoes that can be quantified. Many possible features have been investigated,[26] but in the field of clinical cardiology most progress has been made in the field of analysing one of the simplest: regional echo amplitude.

Echoes arising from the heart may be specular or back-scattered. Specular echoes are generated when the target is large compared with the wavelength of ultrasound used. Their amplitude depends critically on the angle between the reflecting surface and the incident ultrasound beam and is greatest when the two are perpendicular. Examples are those derived from valve cusps or endocardium. Backscattered echoes arise when the targets are small compared with the ultrasound wavelength, and their amplitude is insensitive to their orientation to the ultrasound beam. Myocardium itself is imaged mainly by backscattered echoes; their insensitivity to beam orientation becomes apparent when one considers that on apical views virtually no left ventricular structure is perpendicular to the ultrasound beam, yet the cavity outline can usually be appreciated. The amplitude of backscattered echoes is determined in large part by the stiffness of the structures giving rise to them. Since the Young's modulus of collagen is approximately one thousand times that of myocardium, one would expect regions of scarring to give rise to increased echo amplitude. This has been confirmed qualitatively using M-mode echocardiography[27] and more recently demonstrated to apply quantitatively in man, with echo amplitude correlating with myocardial hydroxyproline concentration.[28]

If measurements of regional echo amplitude are to be made in man, a number of precautions must be observed. Current echocardiographs are constructed by their manufacturers to generate pleasing images, rather than designed as measuring instruments. They frequently contain differentiating and automatic gain compensating circuits as well as a series of post-processing controls which make trivial alterations in the subjective qualities of the image. Any approach to tissue characterization thus needs a radically different outlook. Circuits causing arbitrary changes in amplitude must be inactivated. Ideally, the input-output relation of the echocardiograph should be objectively determined. Depth compensation must be standardized; we have used a standard slope of 2 dB/cm across the image. The master gain setting must also be standardized so that values can be compared from case to case. A practical method is to take the parietal pericardium posterior to the left ventricular wall as an internal standard, and routinely set the master gain so that it is just imaged as a continuous line at the highest grey scale level. We have also used colour to display regional differences in echo amplitude, since this can be more easily appreciated (except by the colour blind), and is not subject to the psychological problems besetting grey scale interpretation. Simple colour substitution degrades the image, so that a system of encoding is used such that grey scale and colour are combined. This runs in real time, allowing instrument gain to be standardized as the recording is being made.[29] Using such an approach, a clear relation between collagen content and myocardial echo intensity can be demonstrated over a very wide range of values (Fig. 3). This method allows myocardial fibrosis to be demonstrated in a number of conditions including ischaemic heart

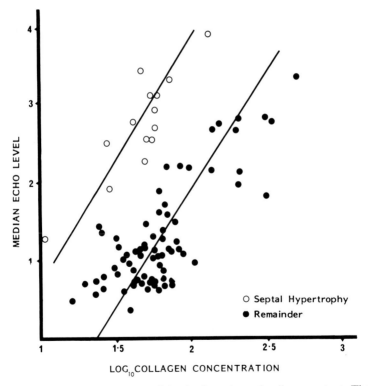

Fig. 3 Relation between myocardial echo intensity and collagen content. The calibration curve of the septum differs from that of the papillary muscles and posterior wall on the parasternal long axis view, probably because it is nearer to the transducer (Reproduced from British Heart Journal 28)

disease, left ventricular hypertrophy, and myocardial involvement associated with eosinophilia.

Myocardial fibrosis significantly affects ventricular function. Papillary muscle involvement leads to mitral regurgitation. In left ventricular hypertrophy, myocardial echo amplitude is independent of left ventricular mass, but correlates closely with abnormalities of diastolic function including prolongation of isovolumic relaxation, and a reduced rate of dimension increase during filling. In addition, echo amplitude is consistently increased when the left ventricular hypertrophy is associated with the T wave changes of left ventricular 'strain'. In eosinophilic heart disease, increased myocardial echo amplitude in the subendocardial region is associated with a restrictive filling pattern, and papillary muscle involvement leads to severe mitral or tricuspid regurgitation.

Oedema is a second possible way in which myocardial stiffness might be increased. In an animal model of unmodified cardiac rejection in the dog both right and left ventricular pixel counts increase strikingly in parallel with the severity of rejection as assessed by histology. In man, striking changes in echo amplitude occur with acute rejection. Plate 14 shows the change over two days in such a patient, in whom septal echo intensity has increased by 15–20 dB. As cyclosporine is used more extensively, however, such episodes have become rare, the usual clinical problem being one of low grade rejection. Nevertheless, such changes can be reliably detected as an increase in echo amplitude, with acceptable specificity and sensitivity compared with endomyocardial biopsy.[30] As with left ventricular hypertrophy, so the increase in echo amplitude associated with rejection is associated with changes in diastolic left ventricular function. These are characteristic, and consist of a reduction in isovolumic relaxation time and an increase in flow deceleration at the end of the period of rapid filling. Their exact cause is not clear, but they probably reflect changes in the passive distensibility of the cavity.

A third potential field of applying these methods is to take account of the observation that myocardial echo amplitude changes throughout the cardiac cycle, increasing by 4–5 dB during ejection.[31] Experimentally, these changes are abolished, along with mechanical activity by coronary artery occlusion. They appear to be more closely related to changes in volume rather than wall tension. They also vary across the myocardium between endo- and epicardium, and so raise the possibility that it might be possible to study function at different levels within the myocardium in intact man.

Clinical echocardiographic tissue characterization is a relatively new field of investigation, and many problems remain to be solved. Estimates of even simple variables such as regional echo amplitude have relatively poor reproducibility. These discrepancies are due in part to uncertainties in standardizing machine gain, patient orientation and path length. In addition, cardiac motion makes it difficult to sample identical regions on successive occasions. Further problems arise when a suitable standard of comparison is sought. For example, histological and biochemical estimates of fibrosis agree only poorly,[28] reflecting their measuring two quite different aspects of a biological process. Echocardiography which measures a third, agrees more closely with biochemistry rather than histology. Problems in identifying a suitable standard of comparison for less well defined entities, such as 'reversible ischaemia' or 'infarct size' are obvious. Perhaps the major problem is lack of knowledge on basic mechanisms of image generation by ultrasound, and of image degradation by passage through proximal tissues.

Cross sectional echocardiography has thus proved of considerable clinical value in detecting the major disturbances of overall and regional ventricular function that occur with disease. Subjective analysis is certainly as satisfactory as that based on contrast angiograms. Tissue characterization allows structural and functional abnormalities to be detected within the myocardium itself, thus providing information inaccessible to standard invasive methods. The potential for future development is considerable; improved image quality, automatic boundary recognition allowing comprehensive documentation of disturbances of timing as well as amplitude, and increased understanding of the relation between myocardial structure and function. Taken with the noninvasive nature of the method, its relative cheapness compared with other imaging methods, its real time applicability and its versatility, the future of these approaches based on ultrasound is obviously secure.

REFERENCES

1 Braunwald E, Ross Jr J, Sonnenblick EH. Mechanisms of contraction in the normal and failing heart. N Engl J Med 1967; 277: 1012–1022
2 Mercier JC, DiSessa TG, Jarmakani JM et al. Two dimensional echocardiographic assessment of left ventricular volumes and ejection fraction in children. Circulation 1982; 65: 962–969

3 Folland ED, Parisi AF, Moynihan PF, Jones DR, Feldman CL, Tow DE. Assessment of left ventricular ejection fraction and volumes by real-time two-dimensional echocardiography. A comparison of cineangiographic and radionuclide techniques. Circulation 1979; 60: 760–766

4 Silverman NH, Schiller NB, Yaeger RL, Ports TA. Left ventricular volume analysis by two dimensional echocardiography in children. Circulation 1980; 548–557

5 Schiller NB, Acquatella H, Ports TA et al. Left ventricular volume from paired biplane two-dimensional echocardiography. Circulation 1979; 60: 547–555

6 Bamber JC, Daft C. Adaptive filtering for reduction of speckle in ultrasonic pulse-echo images. Ultrasonics 1986; 5: 41–44

7 Massay RJ, Logan Sinclair RB, Edmonds J, Bamber JC, Gibson DG. Quantitative effects of speckle reduction on cross sectional echocardiographic images (abstract). Circulation 1987; 76: IV-44

8 Stamm RB, Carabello BA, Mayers DL, Martin RP. Two dimensional echocardiographic measurement of left ventricular ejection fraction: prospective analysis of what constitutes an adequate determination? Am Heart J 1982; 104: 136–144

9 Grant RP. Notes on the muscular architecture of the left ventricle. Circulation 1965; 32: 301–308

10 Gibson DG, Brown DJ. Continuous assessment of left ventricular shape in man. Br Heart J 1975; 37: 904–910

11 Weyman AE, Peskoe SM, Williams ES, Dillon JC, Feigenbaum H. Detection of left ventricular aneurysms by cross-sectional echocardiography. Circulation 1976; 54: 936–944

12 Haendchen RV, Wyatt HL, Maurer G et al. Quantitation of regional cardiac function by two dimensional echocardiography. I. Contraction patterns in the normal ventricle. Circulation 1983; 67: 1234–1245

13 Shapiro E, Marier DL, St John Sutton MG, Gibson DG. Regional non-uniformity of wall dynamics in the normal left ventricle. Br Heart J 1980; 45: 264–270

14 Kronik G, Slany J, Mosslacher H. Die beurteilung der regionalen myokard-funktion im schnittbildechokardiogramm. Z. Kardiol 1980; 69: 92–99

15 Hecht HS, Taylor R, Wong M, Shah PM. Comparative evaluation of segmental asynergy in remote myocardial infarction by radionuclide angiography, two dimensional echocardiography, and contrast ventriculography. Am Heart J 1981; 101: 740–749

16 Ohuchi Y, Kuwako K, Umeda T, Machii K. Real-time, phased-array, cross-sectional echocardiographic evaluation of left ventricular asynergy and quantitation of left ventricular function. Jpn Heart J 1979; 21: 1–15

17 Nixon JV, Narahara KA, Smitherman TC. Estimation of myocardial involvement in patients with acute myocardial infarction by two-dimensional echocardiography. Circulation 1980; 62: 1248–1255

18 Visser CA, Kan G, Lie KI, Becker AE, Durrer D. Apex two dimensional echocardiography: alternative approach to quantification of acute myocardial infarction. Br Heart J 1982; 47: 461–467

19 Moynihan PF, Parisi AF, Feldman CL. Quantitative detection of regional left ventricular contraction abnormalities by two dimensional echocardiography. I. Analysis of methods. Circulation 1981; 63: 752–760

20 Garrison JB, Weiss JL, Maughan WL et al. Quantifying regional wall motion and thickening in two dimensional echocardiograms with a computer-aided contouring system. Proceedings: Ostrow H, Ripley K eds, Computers in Cardiology. IEEE, Long Beach, California, 1977; pp. 25

21 Garcia E, Gueret P, Bennett M et al. Real time computerization of two-dimensional echocardiography. Am Heart J 1981; 101: 783–792

22 Skorton DJ, McNary CA, Child JS, Newton FC, Shah PM. Digital image

processing of two dimensional echocardiograms; identification of the endocardium. Am J Cardiol 1981; 48: 479–486

23 Gibson DG, Brown DJ, Logan-Sinclair RB. Analysis of regional left ventricular wall movement by phased array echocardiography. Br Heart J 1978; 40: 1334–1338

24 Vogel JA, Bastiaans OL, Roelandt J, Honkoop J. Structure recognition and data extraction in two-dimensional echocardiography. In: Lancee C ed. Echocardiology. The Hague: Martinus Hijhoff, 1979; pp. 457–467

25 Gibson D, Mehmel H, Schwarz F, Li K, Kubler W. Changes in left ventricular regional asynchrony after intracoronary thrombolysis in patients with impending myocardial infarction. Br Heart J 1986; 56: 121–130

26 Hill CR. Tissue characterisation. In: Kurjak A ed. Progress in Medical Ultrasound. Amsterdam: Excerpta Medica 1981; 2: pp. 19–25

27 Rasmussen S, Corya BC, Feigenbaum H, Knoebel SB. Detection of myocardial scar tissue by M-mode echocardiography. Circulation 1978; 57: 230–237

28 Shaw TRD, Logan-Sinclair RB, Surin C et al. Relation between regional echo intensity and myocardial connective tissue in chronic left ventricular disease. Br Heart J 1984; 51: 46–53

29 Logan-Sinclair RB, Wong CM, Gibson DG. Clinical application of amplitude processing of echocardiographic images. Br Heart J 1981; 45: 621–627

30 Swanson KT, Greenbaum RA, Logan-Sinclair RB, Gibson DG. Quantitative echocardiographic tissue characterisation after cardiac transplantation. Br Heart J 1988; 59: 629

31 Wickline SA, Thomas III LJ, Miller JG, Sobel BE, Perez JE. The dependence of myocardial ultrasonic integrated backscatter on contractile performance. Circulation 1985; 72: 183–192

British Medical Bulletin (1989) Vol. 45, No. 4, pp. 1076–1091
© The British Council 1989

Colour flow mapping in cardiology: Indications and limitations

G R Sutherland
A G Fraser
Department of Echocardiography, Thoraxcenter, Erasmus University Rotterdam, Rotterdam, The Netherlands

Colour flow mapping (CFM) produces a two-dimensional representation of blood flow within the heart and great vessels by analysing data acquired from multiple pulsed Doppler sample volumes, and displaying mean velocity and turbulence of flow at each site. Constraints imposed by the time required to process these data mean that CFM cannot be used for precise velocity measurements. Instead it depicts flow patterns in healthy and abnormal hearts and the precise location and direction of turbulent jets. CFM is an integral part of the standard echocardiographic examination; it is especially useful in neonates and children with congenital heart disease, and in adults for the semi-quantitative assessment of valve regurgitation, and the description of flow patterns in complex acquired disease. Transoesophageal echocardiography with CFM is invaluable for the diagnosis of mitral prosthetic valve dysfunction, aortic dissection, and complications of infective endocarditis. Intraoperative epicardial CFM provides the equivalent of intraoperative angiography.

Since colour flow mapping was introduced in the early nineteen eighties[1,2] there have been considerable technical advances. The current generation of commercially available systems now produce colour maps of sufficient quality to diagnose a wide range of specific and highly complex flow disturbances. Because these images of abnormal flow patterns within the heart and great vessels are very impressive and easy to understand, ultrasound machines

0007–1420/89/0045–1076/$10.00

which incorporate colour flow mapping are now widely sought by practising cardiologists. It is clear that they provide diagnostic information not obtainable by other techniques.

However, the addition of colour flow mapping to standard duplex scanners remains expensive and the technique has some inherent technical limitations[3] which are perhaps not widely appreciated. This review will describe these limitations, and will indicate the clinical circumstances in which colour flow mapping is of unique value, those in which it provides information complementary to that from standard ultrasound modalities, and those in which it confers little additional benefit over standard duplex scanning. It is hoped that this may allow a prospective purchaser to answer the question: 'Is colour flow mapping a necessary adjunct to my clinical practice or would my money be better spent elsewhere?'

BASIC PRINCIPLES

Colour flow maps are derived from a two-dimensional matrix of pulsed Doppler sample volumes (sometimes as many as 2000 per cross-sectional image). The ultrasound transducer normally used is a standard phased array device with multiple ultrasound crystals aligned at its tip, each emitting an ultrasound beam. Along each beam multiple pulsed Doppler sampling sites are interrogated, thus providing information for analysis which could in theory provide an accurate two dimensional spatial representation of velocities of blood flow. However, so much information returns to the transducer, and the analysis is so complex, that the sampling rate at each site is very low and only mean velocity at each site is calculated. Furthermore, in order to increase the speed of analysis, precise mean velocities are not always calculated. Instead, some machines use the technique known as autocorrelation to analyse the velocity profile along a beam rapidly by comparing it with other profiles acquired from the same direction during other sampling frames. The display is then based on a velocity map produced by analysing changes in velocity over time. Thus in practical terms colour flow mapping systems are essentially mean velocity estimators.

By convention, the colour image is constructed by designating flow towards the transducer at each sampling site in shades of red and flow away from the transducer in shades of blue. Increasing mean velocities towards the transducer are encoded in increasingly lighter (or brighter) shades of red and increasing mean velocities away from the transducer are encoded in lighter shades of blue. In most systems there are 16 shades of either red or blue which can be assigned at each sampling point to display mean velocity. However, the velocity colour map obtained by these means is of limited clinical value. It is only when information on the presence of turbulence is added to the velocity map that colour flow mapping reaches its full potential. Turbulence is recognized on analysis as the presence of a wide variance of velocities of individual blood cells within a particular sampling site. For example, laminar flow has little variation around the mean velocity and a narrow velocity spectrum, so that turbulence will not be detected. On the colour map turbulence is encoded by adding increasing intensities of green to the velocity map, to indicate both the distribution and the intensity of turbulence. In fact, the main value of colour flow mapping systems in the analysis of heart disease is their role as highly sensitive 'turbulence encoders'. All colour flow information is acquired and analysed separately from the cross sectional imaging information. Once both have been processed within the ultrasound machine, the colour flow information is superimposed on the cross-sectional image to create the final display.

In every colour flow system there is a trade off between cross-sectional image quality and the quality of the colour flow map. Normally, image quality is sacrificed to produce an optimal colour flow map. It will be appreciated from the above that the flow information contained within any single colour flow mapping frame is extremely complex. This becomes even more complex when multiple sequential frames are reviewed in real time, for example when a clinical study is reviewed on videotape. In such instances a more detailed analysis may be required to unravel the complexities of the flow disturbance and individual frame by frame analysis may be used.

TECHNICAL LIMITATIONS

Since the frame rate at which colour flow maps are produced is relatively slow (in certain situations this is as little as 8–12 frames per second), imaging during any one cardiac cycle may not demonstrate all flow events which are occurring, particularly if an abnormal jet or area of turbulence is present very transiently or is quite localized, or if the heart rate is fast as in small children. Thus patients should be examined over many cardiac cycles, particularly if there are complex abnormalities of flow, and it may be helpful to record a 'cine loop' of flow events for review frame by frame. When it is difficult to time particular flow events on the real time colour flow map with its slow frame rate, an M-mode colour spectral recording (M–Q mode) may be very helpful as this has a very high sampling rate. This M–Q mode displays the duration and general location of flow events along one selected sampling line within the cross-sectional image, in relation to the electrocardiogram, phonocardiogram, and M-mode echocardiogram.

The maximal mean velocity which can be recorded with colour flow mapping prior to the onset of aliasing is very limited, being just above normal physiological values. Aliasing within the colour map is common, indeed almost universal; it can occur even in normal hearts, for example producing a change of flow colour from red to blue when blood accelerating across the left ventricular outflow tract is viewed in a parasternal long-axis plane. Unlike ordinary pulsed Doppler examinations, in which the peak velocity which can be recorded is increased when the distance between the sample volume and the transducer is reduced, the aliasing limit (Nyquist limit) in colour flow mapping is the same at all sample points along each ultrasound beam. It is determined by the distal limit of imaging, and can therefore be increased only by reducing the depth of field, or to a lesser extent by increasing the pulse repetition frequency. Very occasionally it may be helpful to offset the baseline of the colour spectral display in order to demonstrate a particular area of high velocity flow in more detail. Most importantly, the quality of the colour flow map is always considerably enhanced by narrowing the width of the sector which is scanned, thereby increasing the sampling frame rate.

It follows from these considerations that colour flow mapping cannot accurately measure the mean velocity of abnormal high velocity flows, and is best at demonstrating the site and direction of turbulent flow or any abnormal site or direction of laminar flow, as long as the width of the flow jet is greater than 2 mm.[4] It does not, and for technical reasons cannot, supplant continuous wave or pulsed Doppler techniques for the detailed analysis of either peak velocities or velocity waveforms. Instead, colour flow mapping is excellent for the initial recognition or identification of unexpected or unusual flow patterns, which can subsequently be interrogated using conventional Doppler techniques. It is unique in its ability to demonstrate multiple abnormal jets within the one cardiac chamber. It saves time during a routine Doppler examination by quickly demonstrating abnormal or eccentric jets. The relative strengths of the different Doppler modalities are compared in Table 1.

Since colour flow mapping is not used to measure velocities accurately, the exact alignment of the ultrasound beam with the direction of flow is relatively unimportant when the technique is used to detect abnormal flow, but it should be recognized that the colour which is assigned to a particular jet may change as the angle at which that jet is interrogated is altered. Turbulent flow is easy to detect with colour flow mapping even when the ultrasound source is almost at right angles to flow, because eddies in the vicinity of a turbulent jet are moving in all directions. However, the area of turbulence displayed during colour flow mapping (corresponding for example to the area of a valvar regurgitant jet) is influenced by the overall gain settings used. Normally, very low velocities are not assigned any colour on the colour flow map, and so a regurgitant area may be greatly reduced in size if low gain is used and the ultrasound source is poorly aligned with flow. In general, the colour Doppler gain should be set as high as is possible without producing undue distortion or speckling.

STANDARD COLOUR DOPPLER EXAMINATION

For optimal colour flow images, the ultrasound beam should be directed towards and thus aligned with the flow to be interrogated. Thus in adults, for example, the mitral valve orifice is examined best from an apical four-chamber view and the tricuspid valve from the apical four-chamber view or a parasternal short axis view. Flow across the atrial septum, and in the hepatic veins or inferior vena cava, is best seen from an epigastric sub-xiphoid approach. Flow in the right ventricular outflow tract, across the pulmonary valve and in the main pulmonary artery is seen well from a parasternal short axis study, and flow in the left ventricular outflow tract and across the aortic valve from an apical five-chamber view. In adults, flow in

Table 1 Relative qualities of different Doppler ultrasound modalities

	CFM	PD	CW
Speed of detection of abnormal flow	+ + +	+	+ +
Mapping of abnormal jets	+ + +	+ +	0
Measurement of peak velocity of abnormal flow	0	+	+ + +
Precise evaluation of low velocity waveforms	0	+ + +	+

(CFM = colour flow mapping, PD = pulsed Doppler, CW = continuous wave Doppler; + + + very useful, + + good but more slow, + possible in some circumstances but technical limitations, 0 not possible)

the aortic arch, descending aorta, and pulmonary veins can be seen with colour Doppler imaging from the oesophagus, and in children flow in the aorta or ductus arteriosus can be seen from an infraclavicular or suprasternal approach.

NORMAL COLOUR DOPPLER FINDINGS

In healthy subjects with a normal heart rate and cardiac output, flow within the heart and great vessels is laminar. Aliasing within the colour flow map can occur in localized areas where blood accelerates, for example across the mitral valve orifice or the left ventricular outflow tract, but normally turbulence is not seen, except just next to the tip of a valve leaflet. Transient 'physiologic' regurgitation can occur to a varying degree across all four heart valves, as a normal event at the time of valve closure, and it may be most marked in physically fit young adults with slow heart rates.[5] Frequently, physiologic regurgitation is well demonstrated with colour flow mapping. It seems that all normal subjects have a trace of pulmonary regurgitation, producing a short, low velocity laminar jet,[6] and tricuspid regurgitation is demonstrated so readily that the technique has been described as oversensitive.[7] However, the phenomenon is real, so it is better to state clearly that a trivial whiff of regurgitation is normal. Nevertheless, its detection and localization are facilitated by colour mapping, and even a very small regurgitant jet can then be interrogated with continuous wave Doppler, for example to allow pulmonary artery pressure to be estimated accurately.[8]

CLINICAL APPLICATIONS

Initially, it was thought that the principal application of colour flow mapping would be as an excellent and reliable means of detecting and quantifying valve regurgitation non-invasively.[9] Colour flow mapping is indeed very sensitive at detecting regurgitation,[10] as illustrated in Plate 15, but it is now appreciated that the technique is less good at quantifying it, because the area of turbulence on a flow map associated with a regurgitant jet is determined in part by factors other than the severity of regurgitation; these are discussed below. Instead, it is thought that colour flow mapping is most valuable when characterizing unusual or unexpected flow abnormalities. Some of its major uses are summarized in Table 2. Excellent texts containing recent reviews of these

Table 2   Indications for colour flow mapping

CFM very useful	CFM helpful	CFM of little value
Adults:		
Jet detection and ultrasound alignment for precise CW interrogation	Valve regurgitation (semiquantitation)	Left ventricular function studies
	Left ventricular outflow tract obstruction	Chronic ischaemic heart disease
Post-infarct VSD		Aortic stenosis
LV pseudoaneurysm	Hypertrophic cardiomyopathy	Mitral stenosis
Complex shunting		Pulmonary stenosis
Infective endocarditis		
Aortic dissection		
Prosthetic valve dysfunction (TEE)		
Children/congenital heart disease:		
Neonates/ complex disease	ASD	
Multiple VSD's	Benign murmurs	
Patent ductus arteriosus		
Peripheral pulmonary arterial stenosis		
Both adults and children:		
Intraoperative echocardiography		

(TEE = transoesophageal echocardiography, CW = continuous wave, VSD = ventricular septal defect, ASD = atrial septal defect)

applications have been published, and should be consulted for more detailed accounts of colour flow mapping in particular circumstances.[3,11,12]

In adults, apart from patients with valvar regurgitation, colour flow mapping is of particular value in assessing acute problems such as acquired ventricular septal defect,[13] ventricular pseudoaneurysm,[14,15] or rupture of a papillary muscle, complicating acute myocardial infarction. Combined with transoesophageal cross-sectional imaging, it is useful in a wide variety of conditions,[16,17] many of which have still only been described in case reports. Colour flow mapping is an excellent technique for diagnosing complications of infective endocarditis, such as valve perforation,[18] or fistulae and abscesses.[19] It greatly aids in the diagnosis of acute aortic dissection and can demonstrate details such as flow through an intimal tear or within the true and false lumens.[20,21] It is invaluable in the assessment of prosthetic mitral and tricuspid valve function. Colour flow mapping has been used to diagnose rupture of a sinus of Valsalva aneurysm.[22]

Colour flow mapping is now an essential, integral part of the echocardiographic assessment of neonates and children with congenital heart disease,[23] especially when there is complex shunting. It greatly speeds up investigation, and improves the diagnostic sensitivity of standard duplex scanners in many conditions. Since it is non-invasive, when combined with other echocardiographic modalities it allows the accurate diagnosis of congenital problems in neonates without recourse to cardiac catheterisation and angiography with their inherent risks.[24] Corrective surgery can often be planned on the basis of cross-sectional imaging, spectral Doppler and colour flow data alone.

VALVULAR HEART DISEASE

In general, colour flow mapping provides little additional information about acquired stenotic valvular disease, when compared with continuous wave Doppler. For example in mitral stenosis the jet is usually central so that good alignment of the continuous wave beam is not difficult, but estimates of the peak velocity of mitral stenotic flow are nevertheless more accurate when colour flow mapping is used to provide angle corrections when indicated.[3] Colour flow mapping is a poor technique for the examination of aortic stenotic jets, particularly when the valve is heavily calcified. However, it is a useful technique for the localization of left ventricular outflow tract obstruction, since the distribution of turbulence on the flow map allows differentiation between valvar and sub-valvar obstruction, for example in patients with subaortic membranes.[25] This can sometimes be difficult with imaging alone. In hypertrophic cardiomyopathy it can demonstrate obstruction at apical, midcavity and outflow tract levels.[26] In addition colour flow mapping can clearly identify the sites of right ventricular outflow tract obstruction, for example due to dynamic constriction of the infundibular segment in association with valvar pulmonary stenosis.

The area of turbulence produced on a colour flow map by a valvar regurgitant jet is influenced by many factors.[27] These include not only technical factors such as colour gain settings and the orientation of the ultrasound beam, as already mentioned, but also anatomical and haemodynamic factors. For example in mitral regurgitation the area is affected by the size and configuration of the regurgitant valve orifice, the size of the left atrium, the instantaneous pressure difference between the left atrium and the left ventricle, and the regurgitant jet volume.[3] Such factors are related directly or indirectly to the severity of the regurgitation, but other independent variables such as the loading conditions of the left ventricle and the heart rate also influence the regurgitant area on the flow map. Even when these factors are kept constant in experimental models, it appears that the area of a mitral regurgitant jet is inversely related to the regurgitant orifice area, rather than proportional to it, since the area of a turbulent jet increases if the regurgitant jet velocity is increased.[27] The minimum variability associated with the measurement of a regurgitant jet area by colour flow mapping is about 15%.[28] It has been suggested that such variability is least in mitral regurgitation.[29]

At present, no reliable simple index of severity of regurgitation is available from colour flow mapping. Jet planimetry alone is not adequate for accurate quantification. In clinical studies the closest correlation with angiographic grading of regurgitation is obtained in aortic regurgitation, by measuring the width or cross-sectional area of turbulence produced by the regurgitant jet within the left ventricular outflow tract just below the aortic valve, using a short axis colour flow map and relating this to the area of the left ventricular outflow tract.[30] This approach has also been validated by in vitro studies, which showed that these indices accurately predicted regurgitant fraction even when the aortic diastolic pressure was low.[31] The lateral resolution of the technique was 3 mm. In mitral regurgitation, the best method of quantification described so far, relates the maximal jet area (assessed from orthogonal planes) to the left atrial area.[10] Using such methods, the quantitation of aortic or mitral regurgitation by colour flow mapping is probably at least as reliable as the standard qualitative angiographic assessment, which itself has major limitations. Thus it is unreasonable to criticize only colour flow mapping and standard Doppler techniques for failing to achieve absolute sensitivity and specificity, or precision. Further studies may refine the measurements available, for example by constructing three-dimensional maps of regurgitant volume which incorporate assessment of the duration and velocity of flow, but the indices which are derived are likely to be complex. Colour flow mapping nevertheless offers some advantages, since it is non-invasive and repeatable, so that sequential measurements can be obtained.[32]

In spite of these reservations, qualitative or semi-quantitative assessment of valve regurgitation by colour flow mapping is frequently helpful in the clinical setting. In mitral valve prolapse, for example, the typical pattern of an eccentric posterolateral or anteromedial regurgitant jet can be identified and is specific for either anterior or posterior leaflet prolapse respectively. This eccentricity however makes it difficult to quantify the regurgitation associated with prolapse.[33] During cardiac surgery, epicardial and transoesophageal colour flow mapping can be used to assess regurgitation before cardiopulmonary bypass and after valve repair.[34] Colour flow mapping is a good technique for assessing tricuspid regurgitation; it is more accurate than contrast echocardiography and correlates well with right ventriculography.[35] Transoesophageal colour flow mapping is an excellent technique for the investigation of regurgitant flow across prosthetic mitral valves.[16] Some information can be obtained with colour flow mapping from the chest wall,[36] but flow masking problems[37] mean that a paraprosthetic leak is often detected only from the oesophageal approach. In some circumstances, colour flow mapping provides details of valve regurgitation which cannot be obtained by other methods (Plate 16).

CORONARY HEART DISEASE

Colour flow mapping is of little value in the assessment of patients with angina pectoris or uncomplicated myocardial infarction, but it is very useful in the diagnosis and management of patients with acute complications after infarction. For example, when combined with imaging it readily differentiates between rupture of a papillary muscle, dilation of the mitral valve orifice, and an acquired ventricular septal defect, as the cause of a new systolic murmur. In post-infarct septal defects it can display complex intra-septal flow patterns with multiple entry or exit points, thus providing information of use to the surgeon which cannot be obtained by any other technique. Colour flow mapping is the investigative method of choice for the diagnosis of external cardiac rupture resulting in left ventricular pseudoaneurysm formation.

CONGENITAL HEART DISEASE

Most large ventricular septal defects can of course be seen with conventional cross-sectional echocardiographic imaging, but colour flow mapping provides new information by demonstrating the pattern of flow across each defect. When right and left ventricular systolic pressures are equal, shunting within the defect is multidirectional, and may be seen during diastole as well as systole.[23]

There may be little flow across even quite large non-restrictive defects, if right and left ventricular pressures are equalized, for example when there is coexisting right ventricular outflow tract obstruction. Very small restrictive muscular ventricular septal defects may be undetectable with cross-sectional imaging, but easily identified with colour flow mapping[38] because they produce high velocity turbulent jets, and considerable flow disturbance within the right ventricle. An example of a ventricular septal defect which cannot be seen by cross-sectional imaging but is readily identified by colour flow mapping, is shown in Plate 17. Normally, flow can be seen within the septum itself thus accurately identifying the defect site. Colour flow mapping can also demonstrate multiple ventricular septal defects, although restrictive defects may produce so much turbulence in the right ventricle that individual jets cannot be distinguished, and sometimes more than one jet arises from a single defect. Nevertheless, colour flow mapping is clearly superior in these circumstances to other diagnostic techniques. Its sensitivity for the detection of multiple ventricular septal defects is approximately 70%.[39]

In atrioventricular septal defects colour flow mapping can demonstrate not only shunts across the atrial or ventricular septum, but coexistent mitral or tricuspid regurgitation, or the obligatory shunting from left ventricle to right atrium.[23] In isolated left ventricular outflow tract to right atrial shunting it is the best technique for showing the communication between these chambers. Secundum atrial septal defects can be difficult to see with conventional cross-sectional imaging, because dropout of echo signals from the septum can occur in normal subjects and give rise to confusion, but colour flow mapping can show if there is flow across the atrial septum[40] (Plate 18). It is also helpful for monitoring a Rashkind procedure in neonates with transposition of the great arteries, when it can be used to confirm that an adequate atrial septal defect and shunt has been created. From the oesophagus, colour flow mapping can demonstrate right to left flow across a patent foramen ovale, which appears to be a normal finding in 15% of a healthy population. A sinus venosus atrial septal defect is also well visualized from the oesophageal approach, the morphology of the defect and the co-existing abnormalities of pulmonary venous drainage being clearly demonstrated by the colour flow map.

Colour flow mapping is useful in the diagnosis of patent ductus arteriosus, since it can demonstrate the range of abnormal flow patterns across the duct either directly if the duct is imaged or indirectly when the duct is too small to see, by demonstrating a shunt into the main pulmonary artery.[41] The technique has been used to provide new information about the natural history of ductal flow after birth.[42] Finally, colour flow mapping enhances the echocardiographic detection and description of complex obstruction of the left ventricular outflow tract, for example in children with a sub-aortic membrane,[25] and it allows a precise non-invasive diagnosis of patients with complex lesions associated with continuous murmurs.[43] A discussion of colour flow mapping in more complex congenital heart disease is beyond the scope of this review, but available elsewhere.[23]

INTRA-OPERATIVE ECHOCARDIOGRAPHY

Colour flow maps obtained during cardiac surgery from either an epicardial or a transoesophageal approach can greatly assist the surgeon.[44,45] In some patients the initial study prior to the institution of cardiopulmonary bypass may provide new diagnostic information, but the post-bypass study is of most value. Such early assessment of the functional result of surgery offers the surgeon the chance to reestablish cardiopulmonary bypass to perform further surgery if necessary, and thereby avoid a subsequent operation. For example, significant residual shunts from a previously undiagnosed additional ventricular septal defect, or around the recently inserted patch, can be identified. Our early experience suggests that colour flow mapping is more sensitive than contrast echocardiography at detecting residual shunt flow. The relief of obstruction, for example in subaortic or supra-aortic stenosis, or across the right ventricular outflow tract can be confirmed. Flow through conduits can be assessed, and by using colour flow mapping to align a continuous wave Doppler beam, the pressure gradient produced by banding of the pulmonary artery can be measured. In the switch operation for transposition of the great arteries, it is possible with colour flow mapping to check that the pulmonary arterial and aortic anastomoses are not obstructed. In patients with atrioventricular septal defects the residual atrioventricular valve regurgitation after valve repair can be assessed. Perhaps colour flow mapping is most useful in the intraoperative situation in confirming the successful surgical closure of complex intracardiac shunts, for example from the aorta to the right ventricle.

Intraoperative colour flow mapping is also invaluable in adult patients, for example to assess the results of mitral valve repair operations,[34] but after bypass the regurgitant jet area is very dependent on systolic pressure or left ventricular afterload.[46] It can provide detailed diagnostic information before surgery for aortic dissection,[47,48] and confirm the closure of complex intracardiac fistulae.

CONCLUSIONS

Colour flow mapping is of undoubted benefit in the assessment of congenital heart disease in the neonate, in older children, and during cardiac surgery. In adults, it is of most value in the assessing of abnormal flow patterns in complex acquired heart disease. It assists in the detection and description of valve regurgitation, although it cannot yet be used to quantify regurgitation precisely.

In answer to the original question posed in the introduction to this article, in our opinion colour flow mapping is essential for paediatric cardiologists, and for adult cardiologists working with cardiac surgeons. It is becoming essential for cardiac surgeons, particularly those who operate on patients with congenital heart disease, and it should be available with all transoesophageal echocardiographic systems. It is also valuable to the cardiologist in a general hospital who has a large practice of patients with acute myocardial infarction or valvular heart disease. In all these circumstances colour flow mapping adds significant new information which is not available from other techniques. It clearly has some limitations, but with experience images can be obtained easily which are readily understood and which will assist in clinical decision making.

In our opinion colour flow mapping is a relatively cheap, cost-effective method of investigation which should be available in all the above clinical settings and not just in cardiological 'ivory towers'. It is an everyday practical workhorse in the evaluation of cardiac disease, which once used will never be discarded.

ACKNOWLEDGEMENTS

Dr Fraser holds a British Dutch Fellowship from the British Heart Foundation.

REFERENCES

1 Omoto R, Yokote Y, Takamoto S, et al. The development of real-time two-dimensional Doppler echocardiography and its clinical significance in acquired valvular diseases with special reference to the evaluation of valvular regurgitation. Jpn Heart J 1984; 25: 325–40

2 Bommer WJ, Miller L. Real-time two-dimensional color-flow Doppler: enhanced Doppler flow imaging in the diagnosis of cardiovascular disease. Am J Cardiol 1982; 49: 944 (abstract)

3 Kisslo J, Adams DB, Belkin RN. Doppler color flow imaging. New York: Churchill Livingstone, 1988

4 Tamura T, Yoganathan A, Sahn DJ. In vitro methods for studying the accuracy of velocity determination and spatial resolution of a color Doppler flow mapping system. Am Heart J 1987; 114: 152–8

5 Pollak SJ, McMillan SA, Knopff WD, Wharff R, Yoganathan AP, Felner JM. Cardiac evaluation of women distance runners by echocardiographic color Doppler flow mapping. J Am Coll Cardiol 1988; 11: 89–93

6 Takao S, Miyatake K, Izumi S, et al. Clinical implications of pulmonary regurgitation in healthy individuals: detection by cross-sectional pulsed Doppler echocardiography. Br Heart J 1988; 59: 542–50

7 DePace NL, Ross J, Iskandrian AS, et al. Tricuspid regurgitation: noninvasive techniques for determining causes and severity. J Am Coll Cardiol 1984; 3: 1540–50

8 Hamer HPM, Takens BL, Posma JL, Lie KI. Noninvasive measurement of right ventricular systolic pressure by combined color-coded and continuous-wave Doppler ultrasound. Am J Cardiol 1988; 61: 668–71

9 Sahn DJ. Real-time two-dimensional Doppler echocardiographic flow mapping. Circulation 1985; 71: 849–53

10 Helmcke F, Nanda NC, Hsiung MC, et al. Color Doppler assessment of mitral regurgitation with orthogonal planes. Circulation 1987; 75: 175–83

11 Omoto R. Color atlas of real-time two-dimensional Doppler echocardiography, 2nd Edn. Philadelphia: Lea and Febiger, 1987

12 Houston AB, Simpson IA. Cardiac Doppler ultrasound: a clinical perspective. London: Wright, 1988

13 Zachariah ZP, Hsiung MC, Nanda NC, Camarano GP. Diagnosis of rupture of the ventricular septum during acute myocardial infarction by Doppler color flow mapping. Am J Cardiol 1987; 59: 162–3

14 Roelandt JRTC, Sutherland GR, Yoshida K, Yoshikawa J. Improved diagnosis and characterisation of left ventricular pseudoaneurysm by Doppler colour flow imaging. J Am Coll Cardiol 1988; 12: 807–11

15 Sutherland GR, Smyllie JH, Roelandt JRTC. The advantages of colour flow imaging in the diagnosis of left ventricular pseudoaneurysm. Br Heart J 1989; 61: 59–64

16 Mitchell MM, Sutherland GR, Gussenhoven EJ, Taams MA, Roelandt JRTC. Transesophageal echocardiography. J Am Soc Echo 1988; 1: 362–77

17 Seward JB, Khandheria BK, Oh JK, et al. Transesophageal echocardiography: technique, anatomic correlations, implementation, and clinical applications. Mayo Clin Proc 1988; 63: 649–80

18 Miyatake K, Yamamoto K, Park YD, et al. Diagnosis of mitral valve perforation by real-time two-dimensional Doppler flow imaging technique. J Am Coll Cardiol 1986; 8: 1235–9

19 Fisher EA, Estioko MR, Stern EH, Goldman ME. Left ventricular to left atrial communication secondary to a para-aortic abscess: color flow Doppler documentation. J Am Coll Cardiol 1987; 10: 222–4

20 Iliceto S, Nanda NC, Rizzon P, et al. Color Doppler evaluation of aortic dissection. Circulation 1987; 76: 748–55

21 Takamoto S, Omoto R. Visualization of thoracic dissecting aortic aneurysm by transesophageal Doppler color flow mapping. Herz 1987; 12: 187–93

22 Chia BL, Ee BK, Choo MH, Yan PC. Ruptured aneurysm of sinus of Valsalva: recognition by Doppler color flow mapping. Am Heart J 1988; 115: 686–8

23 Ludomirsky A, Huhta JC. Color Doppler of congenital heart disease in the child and adult. New York: Futura, 1987

24 Reeder GS, Currie PJ, Hagler DJ, Tajik AJ, Seward JB. Use of Doppler techniques (continuous-wave, pulsed-wave, and color flow imaging) in the noninvasive hemodynamic assessment of congenital heart disease. Mayo Clin Proc 1986; 61: 725–44

25 Friedman DM, Schmer V, Rutkowski M. Two-dimensional color Doppler in discrete membranous subaortic stenosis. Am Heart J 1988; 115: 688–91

26 Nishimura RA, Tajik AJ, Reeder GS, Seward JB. Evaluation of hypertrophic cardiomyopathy by Doppler color flow imaging: initial observations. Mayo Clin Proc 1986; 61: 631–9

27 Sahn DJ. Instrumentation and physical factors related to visualization of stenotic and regurgitant jets by Doppler color flow mapping. J Am Coll Cardiol 1988; 12: 1354–65

28 Wong M, Matsumura M, Suzuki K, Omoto R. Technical and biologic sources of variability in the mapping of aortic mitral and tricuspid color flow jets. Am J Cardiol 1987; 60: 847–51

29 Smith MD, Grayburn PA, Spain MG, DeMaria AN, Kwan OL, Moffett CB. Observer variability in the quantitation of Doppler color flow jet areas for mitral and aortic regurgitation. J Am Coll Cardiol 1988; 11: 579–84

30 Perry GJ, Helmcke F, Nanda NC, Byard C, Soto B. Evaluation of aortic insufficiency by Doppler color flow mapping. J Am Coll Cardiol 1987; 9: 952–9

31 Switzer DF, Yoganathan AP, Nanda NC, Woo Y-R, Ridgway AJ. Calibration of color Doppler flow mapping during extreme hemodynamic conditions in vitro: a foundation for a reliable quantitative grading system for aortic incompetence. Circulation 1987; 75: 837–46

32 Otsuji Y, Tei C, Kisanuki A, Natsugoe K, Kawazoe Y. Color Doppler echocardiographic assessment of the change in the mitral regurgitant volume. Am Heart J 1987; 114: 349–54

33 Yoshikawa J, Yoshida K, Akasaka T, Shakudo M, Kato H. Value and limitations of color Doppler flow mapping in the detection and semiquantification of valvular regurgitation. Int J Card Imaging 1987; 2: 85–91

34 Maurer G, Czer LSC, Chaux A, et al. Intraoperative Doppler color flow mapping for assessment of valve repair for mitral regurgitation. Am J Cardiol 1987; 60: 333–7

35 Suzuki Y, Kambara H, Kadota K, et al. Detection and evaluation of tricuspid regurgitation using a real-time, two-dimensional, color-coded, Doppler flow imaging system: comparison with contrast two-dimensional echocardiography and right ventriculography. Am J Cardiol 1986; 57: 811–5

36 Dittrich H, Nicod P, Hoit B, Dalton N, Sahn D. Evaluation of Bjork-Shiley prosthetic valves by real-time two-dimensional Doppler echocardiographic flow mapping. Am Heart J 1988; 115: 133–8

37 Sprecher DL, Adamick R, Adams D, Kisslo J. In vitro color flow, pulsed and continuous wave Doppler ultrasound masking of flow by prosthetic valves. J Am Coll Cardiol 1987; 9: 1306–10

38 Ortiz E, Robinson PJ, Deanfield JE, Kranklin R, Macartney FJ, Wyse RKH. Localisation of ventricular septal defects by simultaneous display of superimposed colour Doppler and cross sectional echocardiographic images. Br Heart J 1985; 54: 53–60

39 Ludomirsky A, Huhta JC, Vick GW, Murphy DJ, Danford DA, Morrow WR. Color Doppler detection of multiple ventricular septal defects. Circulation 1986; 74: 1317–22

40 Suzuki Y, Kambara H, Kadota K, et al. Detection of intracardiac shunt flow in atrial septal defect using a real-time two-dimensional color-coded Doppler flow imaging system and comparison with contrast two-dimensional echocardiography. Am J Cardiol 1985; 56: 347–50

41 Swensson RE, Valdes-Cruz LM, Sahn DJ, et al. Real-time Doppler color flow mapping for detection of patent ductus arteriosus. J Am Coll Cardiol 1986; 8: 1105–12

42 Reller MD, Ziegler ML, Rice MJ, Solin RC, McDonald RW. Duration of ductal shunting in healthy preterm infants: an echocardiographic color flow Doppler study. J Pediatr 1988; 112: 441–6

43 Vargas-Baron J, Attie F, Skronme D, Sanchez-Ugarte T, Keirns C, Santana-Gonzalez A. Two-dimensional echocardiography and color Doppler imaging in patients with systolic-diastolic murmurs. Am Heart J 1987; 114: 1461–6

44 Takamoto S, Kyo S, Adachi H, Matsumura M, Yokote Y, Omoto R. Intraoperative color flow mapping by real-time two-dimensional Doppler echocardiography for evaluation of valvular and congenital heart disease and vascular disease. J Thorac Cardiovasc Surg 1985; 90: 802–12

45 Hagler DJ, Tajik AJ, Seward JB, Schaff HV, Danielson GK, Puga FJ. Intraoperative two-dimensional Doppler echocardiography. A preliminary study for congenital heart disease. J Thorac Cardiovasc Surg 1988; 95: 516–22

46 Czer LSC, Maurer G, Bolger AF, et al. Intraoperative evaluation of mitral regurgitation by Doppler color flow mapping. Circulation 1987; 76: III-108-16

47 Goldman ME, Guarino T, Mindich BP. Localisation of aortic dissection intimal flap by intraoperative two-dimensional echocardiography. J Am Coll Cardiol 1985; 6: 1155–9

48 Omoto R, Takamoto S, Kyo S, Yokote Y. The use of two-dimensional color Doppler sonography during the surgical management of aortic dissection. World J Surg 1987; 11: 604–9

Index

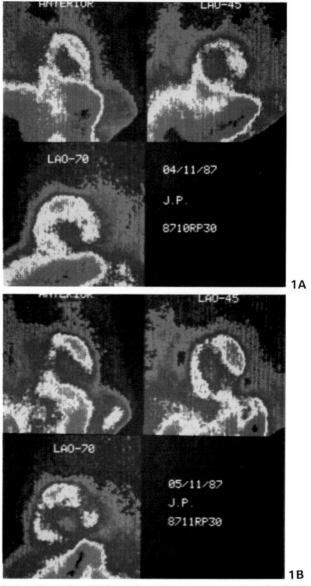

Plate 1A Anterior, 45° and 70° anterior oblique images showing the distribution of technetium 99m-MIBI at rest in a patient with coronary artery disease. Note the problem of splanchnic uptake is considerable with marked overlap onto the inferior wall of the heart. The left anterior oblique 70° image shows a small postero-apical defect. **Plate 1B** Images from the same patient the next day after exercise. The anterior image shows reduced uptake in the distal anterior wall and the apex, the 45° left anterior oblique image shows decreased uptake in the posterolateral wall and apex, and the septum also shows diminished uptake compared to the upper posterolateral wall. The steep left anterior oblique image shows marked tracer reduction in the septum and posterolateral walls compared to the resting images. Note that on exercise splanchnic contribution is much less.

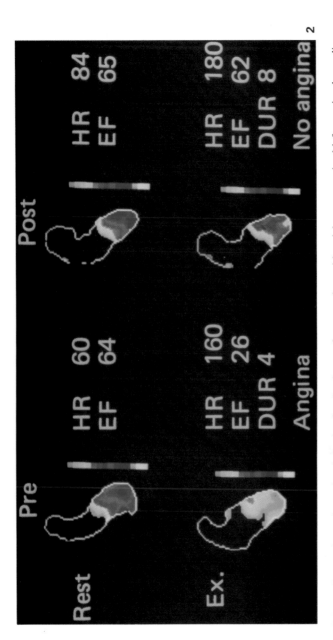

Plate 2 Rest and exercise regional ejection fraction images from a patient with a tight very proximal left anterior descending stenosis, a normal right coronary and circumflex. The two left hand images show the rest and exercise left ventricular function before angioplasty; the two right hand images rest and exercise studies after successful dilation. The regional ejection fraction is represented in a colour scale with yellow and red indicating normal regional function decreasing through purple, green and blue as regional function worsens. It is apparent that resting function is normal both pre and post-angioplasty but all areas of the ventricle show marked dysfunction on exercise (bottom left) before angioplasty with an ejection fraction of 26%. After dilation there is only a very small area of apical hypokinesis and ejection fraction is improved to 62%. A colour bar is shown along side of each image. Abbreviations HR = heart rate, EF = ejection fraction, DUR = duration.

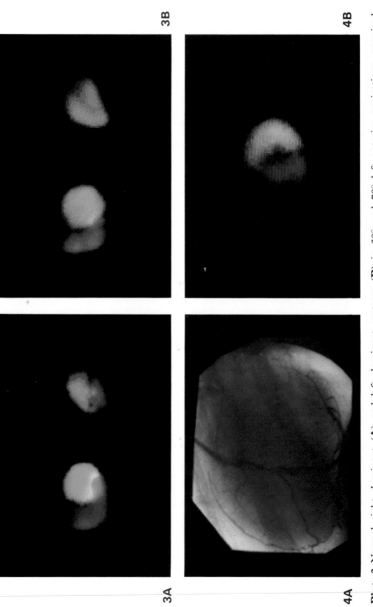

Plate 3 Normal right dominant (**A**) and left dominant systems (**B**) in 30° and 70° left anterior projections, acquired simultaneously, with the right coronary artery injection coded red and the left coronary artery injection coded green. See text for details. **Plate 4A** Coronary angiogram of right coronary artery showing good collateral filling of left anterior descending. **B** Xenon scan in same patient, showing collateral supply to left anterior descending from right coronary artery injection (red). Total occlusion of left anterior descending, with no distribution to septum (left coronary artery injection green)

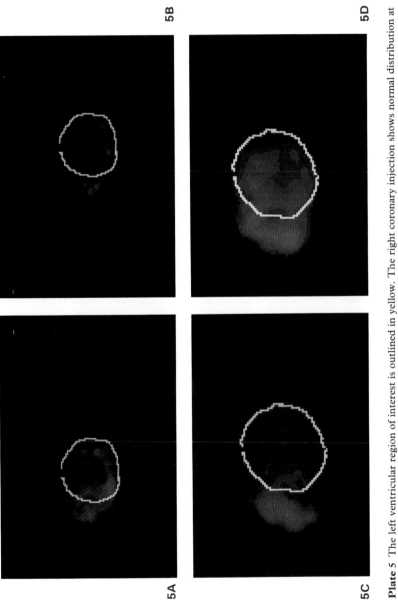

5A

5B

5C

5D

Plate 5 The left ventricular region of interest is outlined in yellow. The right coronary injection shows normal distribution at rest (**A**) which disappears on exercise (**B**). The right coronary injection shows some distribution to the left ventricle, (**C**) but immediately following exercise there is distribution seen to virtually the whole of the left ventricle (**D**).

1099

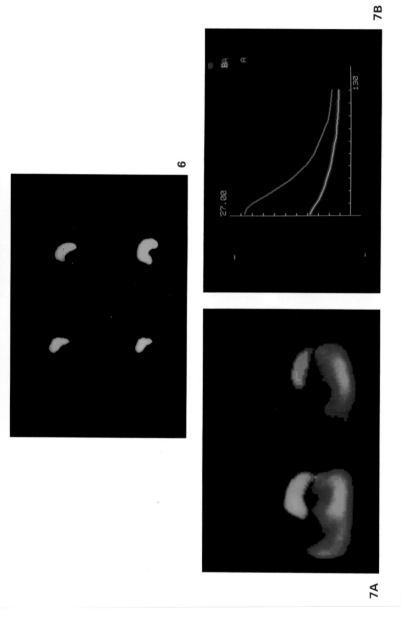

Plate 6 Left intracoronary injection, LHS — Rest injections, RHS — Injection immediately post exercise. Upper panel, control, lower panel 0.4 mg nitrate sublingually for angina at peak exercise. Severe LAD disease, but nitrate increases distribution to left ventricle. **Plate 7A** Left coronary injection, in green. LHS — 30° left anterior oblique and RHS — 70° left anterior oblique projection, in a patient with severe coronary disease. Right coronary artery graft injection, in blue, with distribution to right ventricle and inferior surface of the left ventricle.

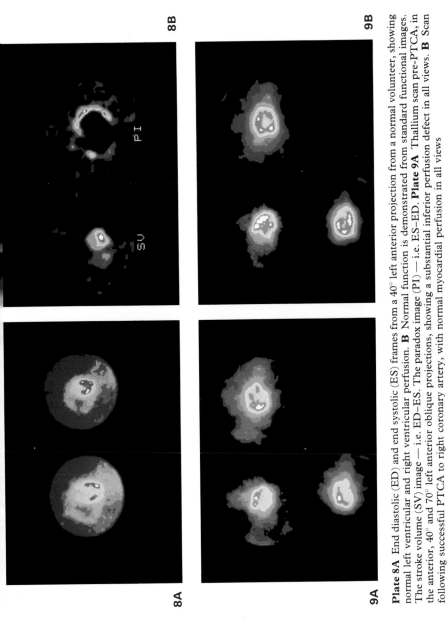

8A

8B

9A

9B

Plate 8A End diastolic (ED) and end systolic (ES) frames from a 40° left anterior projection from a normal volunteer, showing normal left ventricular and right ventricular perfusion. **B** Normal function is demonstrated from standard functional images. The stroke volume (SV) image — i.e. ED−ES. The paradox image (PI) — i.e. ES−ED. **Plate 9A** Thallium scan pre-PTCA, in the anterior, 40° and 70° left anterior oblique projections, showing a substantial inferior perfusion defect in all views. **B** Scan following successful PTCA to right coronary artery, with normal myocardial perfusion in all views

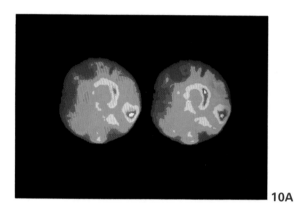

10A

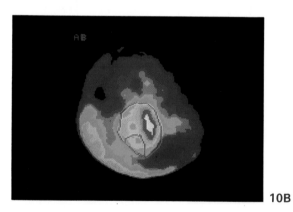

10B

Plate 10A The end diastolic and end systolic frames, in the 40° left anterior projection, showing a substantial anteroapical infarct, in a patient who died within six hours of onset of symptoms. **B** A patient with an inferior infarct, outlined in blue, in the anterior projection, with left ventricular activity outlined in red

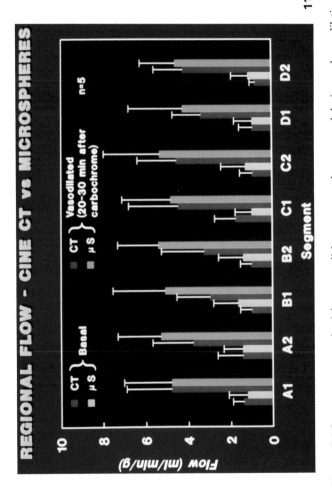

Plate 11 Myocardial flow measurements in eight myocardial segments made at rest and during peak vasodilation induced by carbochrome. Ultrafast CT and radiolabelled microsphere (µS) results are shown at low and high flow states. (Reproduced with permission of Investigative Radiology, Ref. 40 on p. 1010.)

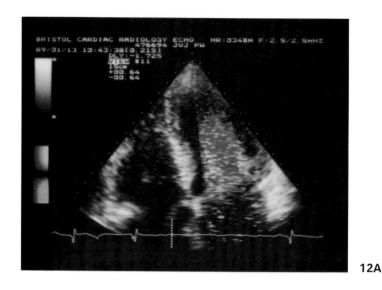

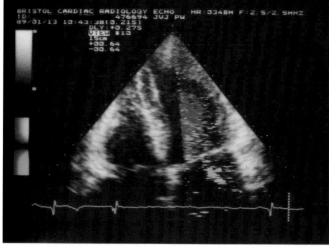

Plate 12 Mitral Regurgitation. (**A**) Colour flow mapping image shows an apical four chamber view. Normal diastolic mitral flow towards the transducer is shown mainly in orange and red tones. (**B**) Systolic view from the same patient. A jet of mitral regurgitation in the left atrium is shown in blue as it moves away from the transducer. Blue tones in the left ventricle show blood moving towards the left ventricular outflow.

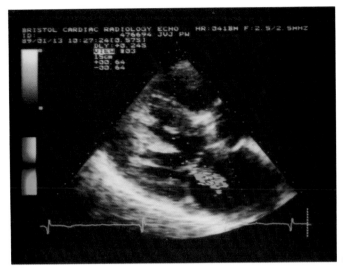

12C

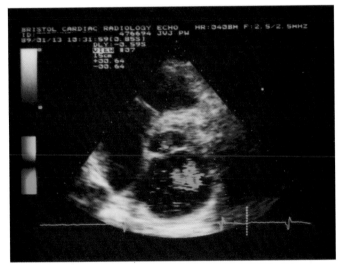

12D

Plate 12 (cont.) (**C**) In the same patient the systolic jet in the left atrium is recorded from the parasternal long axis view. Orange tones within the blue flow are due to aliasing artefact. (**D**) In the same patient the third orthogonal view, the parasternal short axis view, also shows the mitral regurgitant jet (blue) in the left atrium behind the aortic root.

1105

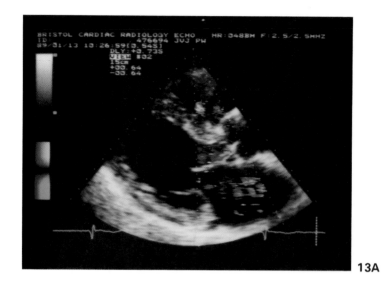

13A

13B

Plate 13 (**A**) Colour flow image showing a parasternal long axis view in a patient with a small diastolic jet of aortic regurgitation (blue). (**B**) In the same patient a short axis view of the left ventricular outflow tract shows the regurgitant jet in cross section.

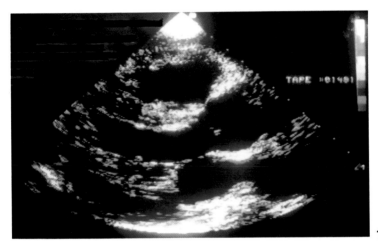

14A

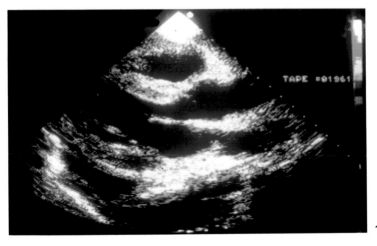

14B

Plate 14A Colour encoded echocardiogram of the left ventricle from a patient early after cardiac transplantation. Echoes of low intensity are imaged as blue or green and of high intensity as blue or white as shown on the colour scale on the right. **B** Echocardiogram recorded with identical gain settings from the same patient two days later, after the appearance of clinical and biopsy evidence of acute rejection. Note the increase in echo intensity, particularly involving the interventricular septum

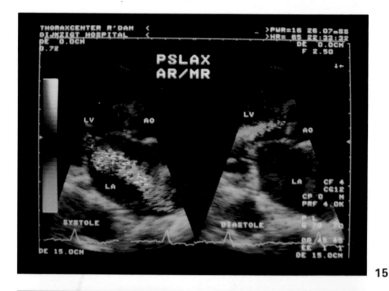

15

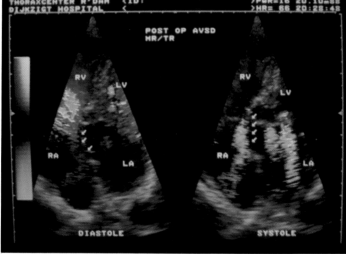

16

Plate 15 Colour flow maps obtained in a standard parasternal long axis plane. The systolic frame demonstrates a turbulent jet of mitral regurgitation extending from the central part of the mitral valve almost to the left atrial posterior wall, and the diastolic frame demonstrates a small regurgitant jet from mild aortic regurgitation. In the diastolic frame pulmonary venous inflow into the left atrium can be seen (in red). Ao = aorta, LV = left ventricle, LA = left atrium. **Plate 16** Colour flow maps obtained from the apex in a 4-chamber view, in a patient studied after surgical repair of an atrioventricular septal defect. The integrity of the atrial septal repair (patch indicated by arrows) is confirmed since there is no shunt across the atrial septum, but the systolic colour map demonstrates tricuspid regurgitation and 2 separate jets of mitral regurgitation. LV, LA as in Plate 15. RV = right ventricle, RA = right atrium.

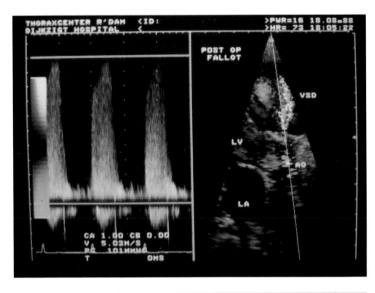

17

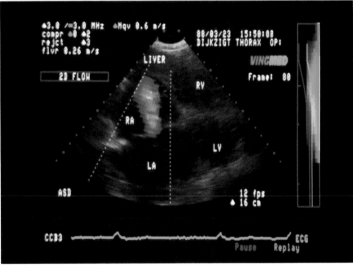

18

Plate 17 Parasternal long axis cross section of the heart in a patient studied after cardiac surgery for the tetralogy of Fallot (right hand frame). During systole, there is a prominent turbulent jet extending into the right ventricle from the area of the septal patch. Interrogation of this jet with continuous wave Doppler (left hand frame) reveals a peak velocity of 5 m/sec, confirming that the residual ventricular septal defect is restrictive. Abbreviations as in Plate 15. **Plate 18** Subxiphoid 4-chamber view, with superimposed colour flow map restricted to the area between the green dotted lines. The laminar flow extending from the interatrial septum anteriorly into the right atrium (shown in red) indicates a non-restrictive atrial septal defect. Abbreviations as in other figures.